The Perrin Technique

This book is dedicated to the two most important ladies in my life

Julie
(My wife and soul-mate)

and

Hilda
(My mother who reached 75 on the day I finished this book)

The Perrin Technique

How to beat chronic fatigue syndrome/ME

Dr Raymond Perrin

DO, PhD
Registered Osteopath
and Specialist in Chronic Fatigue Syndrome

Honorary Senior Lecturer
Department of Allied Health Professions
University of Central Lancashire,
Preston, UK

Research Director of the F.O.R. M.E. Trust

Founder and Clinical Director of the Perrin Clinic™

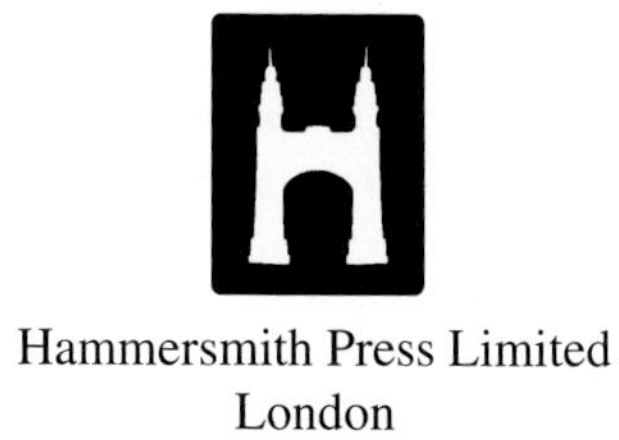

Hammersmith Press Limited
London

First published in 2007 by Hammersmith Press Limited
496 Fulham Palace Road, London SW6 6JD, UK
www.hammersmithpress.co.uk

Whilst the advice and information in this book are believed to be true and accurate at the date of going to press, neither the author nor the publisher can accept any legal responsibility or liability for any errors or omissions that may be made. In particular (but without limiting the generality of the preceding disclaimer) while every effort has been made to ensure that the contents of this book are accurate, it must not be treated as a substitute for qualified medical advice. Neither the author nor the publisher can be held responsible for any loss or claim arising out of the use, or misuse, of the suggestions made or the failure to take medical advice.

British Library Cataloguing in Publication Data: A CIP record of this book is available from the British Library.

ISBN 978-1-905140-12-1

Commissioning editor: Georgina Bentliff
Edited by Anne Charlish
Designed by Julie Bennett
Photography by Stuart Derbyshire (treatment and exercise technique) and the author
Diagrams drawn by Prof. Jim Richards and the author
Typeset by Phoenix Photosetting, Chatham, Kent
Production by Helen Whitehorn, Pathmedia
Printed and bound by TJ International Ltd, Padstow, Cornwall, UK
Cover image: Woman Holding Her Back © JLP/Sylvia Torres/CORBIS

Contents

List of illustrations

Acknowledgement

> Sometimes our light goes out but is blown into flame by another human being. Each of us owes deepest thanks to those who have rekindled this light.
>
> *Albert Schweitzer* (1875–1965)

Throughout the last seventeen years, while I was writing my thesis and this book, there have been many people to whom I owe an enormous debt of gratitude in enabling me to finish my thesis, in July, 2005, and subsequently this book.

I would like to pay tribute to the benefactors, scientists, colleagues, patients, family members, staff and friends who have all played a pivotal role in my years involved with CFS/ME research, culminating in the completion of this publication.

Firstly, I would like to express my heartfelt thanks to The David and Frederick Barclay Trust for providing the funds for this research. Since the establishment of the Fund for Osteopathic Research into ME (FORME) in February 1995, there have been some exceptional members of the public who have served as trustees of FORME. I thank them all, especially vice-chair and founder Riaz Bowmer, as well as past chairmen Darren Mercer and Chris March. My special thanks go to Ruth Behrend, Kelvin Heywood, Steve Briggs and Sue Peers for their continuing funding and support.

Let me extend my thanks, too, to my first CFS/ME success, Pete, who insisted that I begin this long road of research, and my many patients over the years who have contributed advice, encouragement and research funds. I thank Dr C. Royde, a retired Manchester general practitioner, who, in the early days of my research, gave me encouragement and advice from an orthodox medical perspective and checked my earliest work. Thanks also to Dr Anne Macintyre and to Dr Andrew Wright for their invaluable information and inspiration.

Many thanks to Professor Jack Edwards, who initially took me under his wing in my early years at Salford University's Department of Orthopaedic Mechanics, for his patience, guidance and for his meticulous checking of my thesis. Thanks, too, to health psychologist Dr Pat Hartley, joint supervisor with Professor Edwards, for her guidance.

My main supervisor during the research, Dr Vic Pentreath, has been a source of immense support and, without his cajoling, positive advice and cheerful disposition, I might never have persevered.

Let me thank Professors Alan Jackson and Jim Richards, who have both imparted a mere fraction of their practical skills and immense knowledge in neuroradiology and biomechanics respectively, which are incalculably useful.

I am also very grateful to the following:

My colleagues Sophie King and Mark Stern, Darren Hayward, at my London and Manchester clinics for coping with years of organised chaos. My secretary Elaine Coleman for her superb clerical and organisational skills and Melissa for modelling her healthy spine. My patients-turned-models for the photographs in this book. My father Bernard Perrin, and my father-in-law Colin Fretwell, for proofreading my original thesis. My nephew, Simon Klein, for his computer skills.

Thanks go to Shirley Trickett and my publisher Georgina Bentliff who both gave me the final encouragement to finish the book, as well as my editor Anne Charlish, and all the staff at Hammersmith Press for helping to bring my work to a much wider audience.

My sons Jonathan, Max and Joshua all deserve a mention as they have had to do part of their growing up with a dad who was often engrossed in his work. Last, but never least, I must pay tribute to my wife Julie who is a true jewel. Through her own long battle with CFS/ME, Julie has empathised with my patients and patiently supported my work week by week, year by year.

Introduction

My book describes a journey of discovery that started as a consequence of an event in 1989, which some would say was fate, others luck. A simple appointment for back pain led to a former cyclist changing my life forever and helping to improve the lives of countless people around the world. This book has been written as an informative guide for people who suffer from chronic fatigue syndrome (known in Great Britain as CFS/ME), while revealing the trials and tribulations of the innovative research into the disease that led to the formation of The Perrin Technique.

Many ideas have been put forward to explain the cause of chronic fatigue syndrome (CFS/ME) but, as yet, nobody has offered a universally accepted theory that has led to a successful treatment programme. As an osteopath, trained in the manual diagnosis and treatment of the body, I have discovered a probable mechanical cause of the disease. The details of my theory are contained within this book, interspersed with the background story of the research itself.

There was no proof in 1989 for the concept of CFS/ME having physical causes, and thus I have spent some seventeen years researching the medical facts, looking at pathological mechanisms in other conditions, and finding plenty of scientific evidence to validate the concept that mechanical problems may lead to CFS/ME. The results of this research will help you to understand the underlying cause of the disorder.

I have included a comprehensive guide to the manual treatment of CFS/ME that should prove helpful to both practitioner and patient. This fresh approach to fighting the disease will, I hope, improve the health of millions of sufferers throughout the world.

For those readers who are not familiar with all of the medical terms in the book, there is a comprehensive glossary at the end. This should enable the patient, as well as the practitioner, fully to understand my approach and to benefit from treatment for the debilitating condition of CFS/ME.

Raymond Perrin
Manchester, 2007

Chapter 1

How the Perrin Technique works

> Thou shalt make me hear of joy and gladness; that the bones which Thou hast broken may rejoice.
>
> *Book of Psalms LI, verse 10*

Hundreds of patients have visited my practice with signs and symptoms of CFS/ME. All of them share common structural and physical signs, while complaining of strikingly similar symptoms. This cannot be dismissed purely as coincidence.

My theory for the diagnosis and treatment of CFS/ME started with a patient: this case was the first and perhaps the most dramatic of all the CFS/ME patients I have treated. In 1989 an executive, who shall be referred to as Mr E, walked into my city centre practice, in Manchester, where I ran a clinic specialising in treating sports injuries. He had been a top cyclist, racing for one of the premier teams in the Northwest of England.

He had suffered from a recurring, low back pain, which, after examination, I had diagnosed to be a strain of the pelvic joints. While treating his pelvis, I noted that his dorsal spine was particularly restricted. I enquired whether or not he had any problems in his upper back, and he acknowledged that for years, during his cycling, he had experienced a dull ache across his shoulders and at the top of his back. This in itself was nothing significant, as it was very common to find cyclists with pelvic problems and a stiff and bent dorsal spine. What was interesting was the fact that, for the past seven years, Mr E had been diagnosed as suffering from CFS/ME.

Mr E complained of tingling in both hands and a 'muzzy' feeling in his head. He suffered general fatigue and an ache in his knees, as well as the pain in his back and shoulders. He had been forced to stop racing since the onset of the disorder.

This patient was one of many who came to me after being diagnosed by their doctor, or specialist, as suffering from CFS/ME. At that time, although I had helped other patients with CFS/ME, I had done no research into the disease, and I had no specific treatment programme for the disorder.

With only five treatments, Mr E's back was better, but, most incredibly, the signs and symptoms of CFS/ME had drastically improved. He was symptom-free after a mere two months from the start of treatment. He still remains healthy and the last news I heard of him was that he had moved to Holland, cycling with the same power and zeal that he used to enjoy prior to his illness.

It was after helping this patient that I realised that there must be a relationship between the mechanical strain on the thoracic spine and CFS/ME. Although I had not set out to cure the fatigue signs and symptoms in this patient, I had done exactly that by improving the posture and movement in the upper back. My thoughts turned to the other CFS/ME patients that I had treated. The restriction of the dorsal spine was a common factor that could not be ignored.

Professional sportsmen, and people who are keen on sporting events, usually start participating in their discipline at an early age. These competitive individuals are more likely to suffer from developmental disorders commonly associated with overtaxing growing bones and joints.

One such disorder is osteochondritis. This is an inflammatory disorder of the bone and cartilage, which often affects an active, growing spine, and is a frequent cause of backache in adolescents. The disorder usually leaves a slight permanent deformity in the spine, especially in the thoracic area, with an associated restriction of the affected region. This stiffened area may be asymptomatic for the rest of the person's life, but it may lead to other mechanical problems of the back. This condition could eventually cause permanent irritation of the surrounding sympathetic nerves, and thus be a further reason for the high incidence of CFS/ME in active, sporty men and women.

I am now going to summarise my theory of the diagnosis and treatment of CFS/ME. If you don't enjoy reading or, because of CFS/ME you are unable to concentrate on long texts, this one chapter is for you. If, after reading it, you wish to understand what CFS/ME is all about, the rest of the book is waiting to be read. I endeavour to keep the explanations as simple as possible in this first chapter.

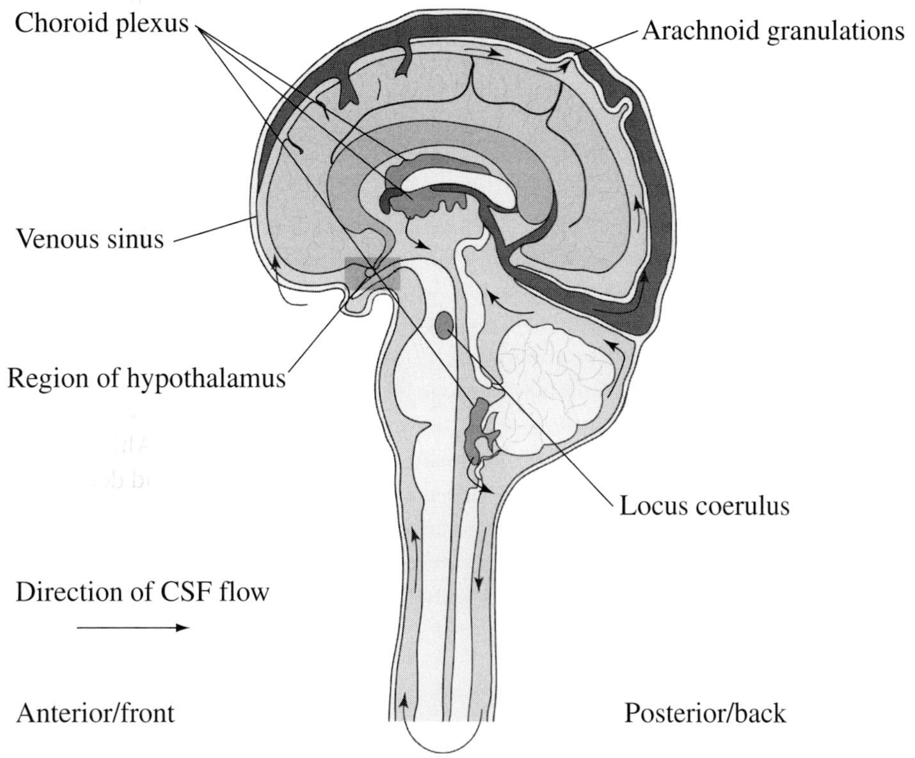

Figure 1. *Flow of cerebrospinal fluid and the position of the hypothalamus.*
The fluid's journey is shown from its production at the choroid plexus around the brain and spinal cord with most of the CSF draining into the venous sinuses. Further drainage takes place via the lymphatics.

Fact 1: Fluid flow

A fluid flows around the brain and continues up and down the spinal cord: this is the cerebrospinal fluid. This fluid has many functions, for example, as a protective buffer to the central nervous system and for supplying nutrients to the brain. However, one function has been known about since the 1860s[1] but has only received significant attention in recent years,[2–15] and that is the drainage of poisons (toxins) out into the lymphatic system.

Fact 2: Getting the toxins out

The lymphatic system is an organization of tubes around the body that provides a drainage system secondary to the blood flow. Why does the body need a secondary system to cope with poisons or foreign bodies in the tissue? Are the veins not good enough? The answer in one important word is 'size'. The blood system does process poisons and particles, but the trouble is that foreign material enters it via the walls of the microscopic blood vessels, known as the capillaries. Their walls resemble a fine mesh, which acts as a filter, thus allowing only small molecules to enter the bloodstream itself. This process is known as filtration. When the blood reaches the liver, detoxification takes place, cleansing the blood of its impurities. The capillary beds of lymphatic vessels, known as terminal lymphatics, take in any size of toxin, via a wall that resembles the gill of a fish, opening as wide as is necessary to engulf the foreign body. These large molecules of toxins often need breaking down before entering the blood stream: and so they begin the process of detoxification in the lymph nodes on the way to drainage points just below the collar bone into two large veins (the subclavian veins), with most of the body's lymph draining into the left subclavian vein (see Fig. 2). Once the toxins have drained into the subclavian veins, they eventually

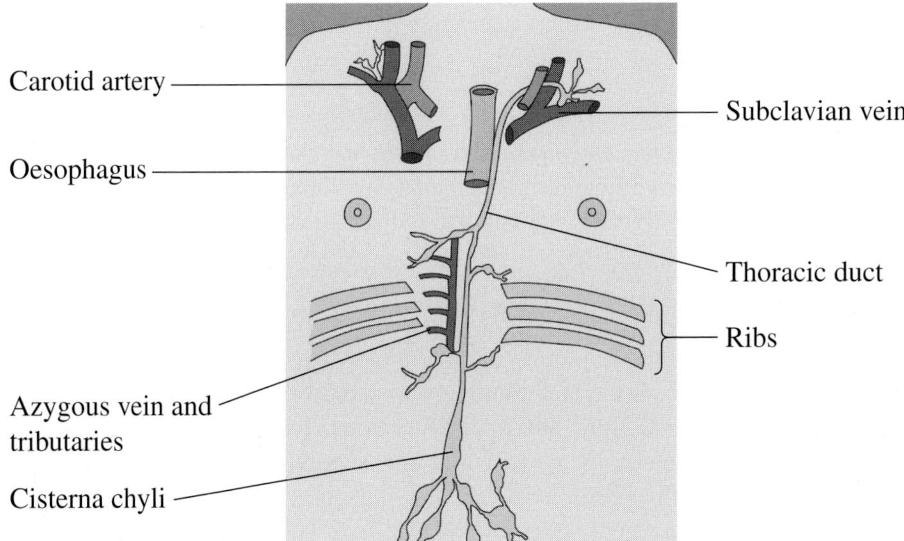

Figure 2. *The thoracic duct (the central lymphatic drainage system into the blood).*

find their way into the liver and, as is the case with normal circulatory toxins, are broken down by the liver[16].

Fact 3: The pumping mechanism

For a long time after it was discovered, the lymphatic system was thought not to have a pump of its own. Its flow was believed to depend on the massaging effect of the surrounding muscle and the blood vessels lying next to the lymphatics, akin to squeezing toothpaste up the tube. However, Professor John Kinmonth, a London chest surgeon, discovered in the 1960s that the main drainage of the lymphatics, the thoracic duct, has a pumping mechanism in its walls[17,18,19] and that this is controlled by the sympathetic nervous system.[20] If there is a disturbance of the sympathetic nervous system, the pump may push the lymph fluid in the wrong direction and lead to a further build-up of toxins in the body.

Fact 4: The sympathetic nervous system

The sympathetic nervous system is part of the autonomic nervous system, which deals with all the automatic functions of the body. The sympathetic nervous system is important in controlling blood flow and the normal functioning of all the organs of the body such as the heart, kidney, and bowel. We know it is vital for healthy lymphatic drainage. In CFS/ME sufferers the sympathetic nervous system will have been placed under stress for many years before the onset of the signs and symptoms of the illness. This stress may be of a physical nature due to postural strain or an old injury, it may be emotional, environmental such as pollution, or it may be due to stress on the immune system due to infection or allergy (Fig. 3).

The sympathetic nerves spread out from the thoracic spine to all parts of the body and are ultimately controlled by a small site in the brain, the hypothalamus (see Fig. 1), which also controls all the hormones of the body.

Fact 5: Biofeedback

The hypothalamus controls hormones by a process called biofeedback. This mechanism can be explained with the following example. If the sugar levels in the body are too low, that may be due to a rise in the hormone insulin, which is produced in the pancreas under control of the hypothalamus. Insulin, like other hormones, is a large protein molecule that travels through the blood and stimulates the breakdown of sugar. It passes from the blood into the hypothalamus, which will calculate if more or less insulin production is required and, accordingly, send a message to the pancreas to make the necessary adjustments.

The region of the hypothalamus is the only section of the brain that allows the transfer of large molecules into the brain from the blood. In all other parts of the brain there is a filter known as the blood-brain barrier, similar to the fine mesh in the small blood vessels mentioned earlier. The blood-brain barrier prevents toxins and other harmful material entering the brain's cells from the blood. However, this barrier is naturally weakened at the hypothalamus to enable the biofeedback mechanism to work and allow the transfer of hormones. Unfortunately, this weakness means that large toxic molecules can invade the brain and wreak havoc on the normal functioning of the central nervous system.[21–26]

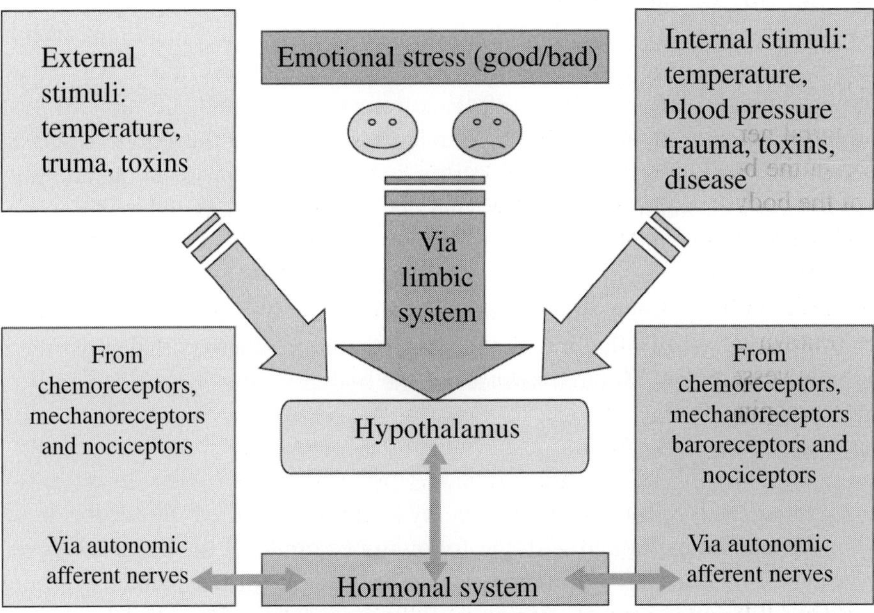

Figure 3. *Long-term build-up of internal and external stress.*

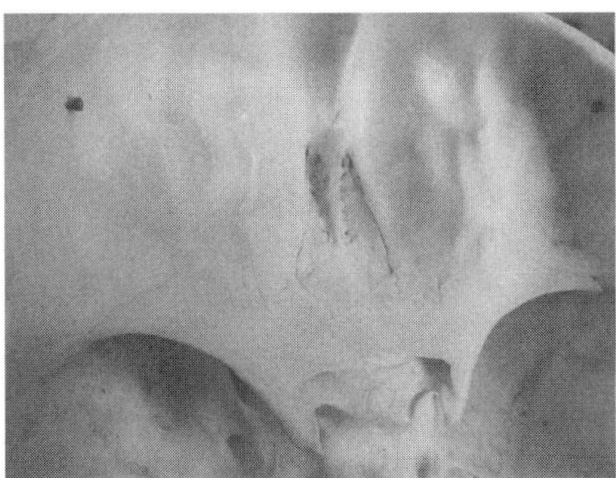

Figure 4. *Superior view of the cribriform plate with observed perforations.*
The perforations seen above allow the passage of blood vessels, nerves and cerebrospinal fluid from the cerebrum to the nasal sinuses situated directly below the ethmoid bone. This drainage problem appears to arise from a prior defect in the skull, usually in the frontal/nasal region due to either a congenital, hereditary or traumatic aetiology. This may be exacerbated by chronic sinusitis, leading to further congestion affecting the lymph channels in the mucous membranes of the nasal sinuses.

Fact 6: What goes wrong

The central nervous system, composed of the brain and the spinal cord, is the only region in the body that has no lymphatic system. The role of the lymphatics in the rest of the body is to capture and process large invading molecules: so what can the central nervous system do if attacked by large toxins? The cerebrospinal fluid (see Fact 1) drains toxins along minute gaps next to blood vessels through perforations in the skull, with the largest amount draining through a bony plate situated above the nose (known as the cribriform plate, Fig. 4).[3,12,14,15] The toxins then drain into lymphatic vessels in the tissue around the nasal sinuses. There is further drainage of the cerebrospinal fluid down the spine and outwards to pockets of lymphatic vessels running alongside the spine.[4,5,7] The lymphatic vessels take the toxins away via the thoracic duct (see Fig. 2) into the blood and the liver where they are broken down.

Fact 7: Build-up of toxins

In CFS/ME it is these drainage pathways, both in the head and the spine, that are not working sufficiently, leading to a build-up of toxins within the central nervous system. The reasons for drainage problems can vary from patient to patient. It may be trauma to the head from an accident, it may be hereditary or due to a problem at birth. The spine may become out of alignment – especially in very active teenagers – which can lead to a disturbance in the normal drainage (Fig 5.). If the spine and brain are both affected, the increased toxicity will reduce hypothalamic function and thus will further affect sympathetic control of the central lymphatic vessel. This in turn pumps more toxins back into the tissues and the brain, which further affects sympathetic control. With this, a vicious circle (see Fig. 6) has started.[27,28,29]

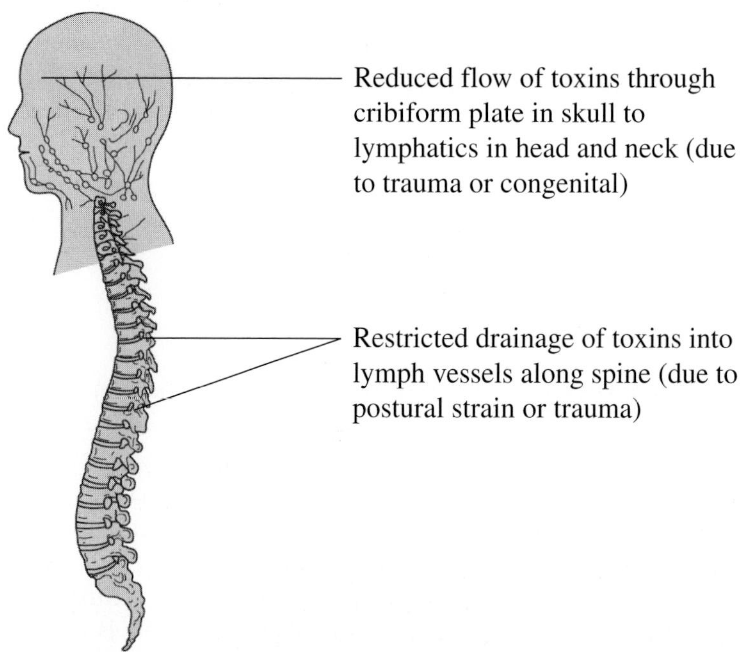

Figure 5. *Restricted drainage of toxins from the central nervous system.*

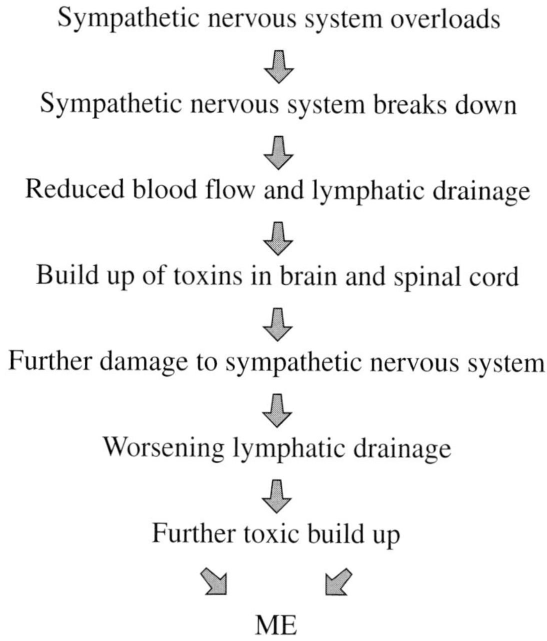

Figure 6. *The downward spiral into CFS/ME.*

Conclusion

CFS/ME is very much a structural disorder with clear and diagnosable physical signs, including disturbed spinal posture, swollen lymph vessels and specific tender points related to sympathetic nerve disturbance and backflow of lymphatic fluid. The fluid drainage from the brain to the lymphatics moves in a rhythm that can be palpated using cranial osteopathic techniques. A trained practitioner can feel a disturbance of the cranial rhythm in CFS/ME sufferers.[29, 30]

The Perrin Technique helps drain the toxins away from the central nervous system and incorporates manual techniques that stimulate the healthy flow of lymphatic and cerebrospinal fluid and improve spinal mechanics. This in turn reduces the strain on the sympathetic nervous system, which aids a return to good health.

Chapter 2

CFS/ME: What it is

Nor bring to see me cease to live
Some doctor full of phrase and fame
To shake his sapient head and give
The ill he cannot cure a name

Matthew Arnold (1822–1888)

Chronic fatigue syndrome affects the communication between the internal organs and the musculoskeletal components of the body. This organ of communication is known as the **sympathetic nervous system**, which may be likened to a transmission system in a power station.

In our homes and at work we use electricity for lighting, for cooking, refrigerating and freezing, for household electrical appliances, and for music centres, TVs and computers. The electrical energy required is produced by power stations and is monitored by controllers in a transmission station, which channels the amount of electricity through to us, the consumers.

If we were all suddenly to use substantially more electricity, simultaneously, the transmission station would allow more electricity to flow, signalling to the power stations to produce more energy. This occurs, for example, at 'halftime', during major international televised sporting events, when everybody turns on the kettle at the same time to make a cup of tea.

If something was wrong with the operator, or the equipment in the transmission station was faulty, the power required to cope with the increased demand would be insufficient. This would eventually lead to a power cut and blackout. Alternatively, if a situation arose when too much electricity passed into the household's supply, an overload or power surge could damage the appliances in use at that time.

In the body, the muscles are the principal 'electrical appliances', utilising most of the energy produced. The power station of the body is the gastro-intestinal system together with the respiratory system, which consumes fuel in the form of food and utilises oxygen to produce the energy.

The sympathetic nervous system is the transmission station, which connects the visceral 'power station' of the body to the musculoskeletal 'appliance'.

Blackout

When we are active, the sympathetic nervous system stimulates an increase of energy production and a release of stored energy. If this is not accomplished, the result is that the muscles will not receive enough of the nutrients normally obtained from the blood, and the natural function of the muscles, nerves and joints will break down. There will be a power cut in our body and we will suffer fatigue.

This is precisely what occurs in patients suffering from CFS/ME. The body demands more energy, especially when under any form of stress, mental or physical. However, the mechanism normally operated to transform the stored energy into a usable form is not functioning, and thus the patient's body simply stops working effectively.

CFS/ME is a profoundly debilitating disorder and requires as much rest as possible to reverse the process by minimising the amount of stress on the body. The power station analogy explains why some sufferers seem to display signs of too much sympathetic activity such as palpitations and excessive sweating as well as reduced sympathetic activity such as fatigue and low blood pressure. The fault with the 'transmission station' can lead to part of the body working in overdrive and another section of the sympathetic nervous system in a power cut scenario. Reducing the demand on the sympathetic nervous system helps the patient on to the road to a full recovery.

What it is called

The disorder CFS/ME is known to many as ME, chronic fatigue syndrome or post-viral fatigue syndrome. In the United States it is now more commonly referred to as chronic fatigue and immune dysfunction syndrome (CFIDS).

Most diseases are classified according to the type of change that takes place in the cells of the body. Some diseases are categorised according to causative factors, e.g. a viral infection or a bacterial infection. The problem with Chronic Fatigue Syndrome (CFS/ME) is that it does not fit into any particular category.

CFS/ME is so diverse in its signs and symptoms that no specific disease classification fits the bill. Thus the term myalgic encephalomyelitis: myalgic refers to pain in muscles and encephalomyelitis relates to the possible effect on the brain and spinal cord. This term may suggest that there is inflammation of the central nervous tissue. However, with CFS/ME, inflammation of the spinal cord is not always present. Although some general practitioners, physicians, rheumatologists and immunologists recognise the category CFS/ME and realise that there is something wrong with the patient, they do not know what to diagnose or how to treat.

Most of my patients who suffer from CFS/ME have been to neurologists, undergone brain scans, X-rays, blood tests and many other exhaustive examinations, all of which have yielded inconclusive evidence. The usual advice given to sufferers is to rest until the body sorts itself out or they may be told to get on with life as best they can and try to forget about it.

How CFS/ME may be defined

Chronic fatigue syndrome (CFS) or myalgic encephalomyelitis (ME), as it has been known in the UK since an outbreak was identified by physician Dr Melvyn Ramsay in 1955 at London's Royal Free hospital,[1] is a clinically accepted condition now referred to in Great Britain as CFS/ME. As the suffix 'itis' means inflammation of some kind, some health professionals now use the term myalgic encephalomyelopathy, signifying a disease state within the spine but not necessarily accompanied by inflammation.

We know that CFS/ME is characterized by:

- generalised abnormal muscle fatigue that occurs after relatively mild activity
- sleep disturbance
- headache
- cognitive dysfunction
- depression
- increased sensitivity to light and sound
- back pain
- neck pain
- sore throat

- irritable bowel
- bladder pain.

The name chronic fatigue syndrome, compared with alternative terms, best describes this illness. The use of the term ME (myalgic encephalomyelitis/myalgic encephalomyelopathy), which is not widely used except in the UK and Canada, can lead to confusion and may substantially undermine the progress that has been made by research to date. The joint term CFS/ME has been agreed upon by the UK's independent working group in its report into the condition to the Chief Medical Officer, published on 11 January 2002,[2] and I believe it to be the most suitable name at present.

CFS, according to Dr Keiji Fukuda and his colleagues[3] at the Centre of Disease Control, Atlanta, USA, in 1994, is defined by the presence of the following:

- clinically evaluated, unexplained persistent or relapsing chronic fatigue that is of new or definite onset (has not been lifelong)
- is not the result of ongoing exertion
- is not substantially alleviated by rest
- results in substantial reduction in previous levels of occupational, educational, social, or personal activities.

In addition, the concurrent occurrence of four or more of the following signs and symptoms must exist, all of which must have persisted or recurred during six or more consecutive months of illness and must not have predated the fatigue:

- self-reported impairment in short-term memory or concentration severe enough to cause substantial reduction in previous levels of occupational, educational, social, or personal activities
- sore throat
- tender cervical or axillary lymph nodes
- muscle pain
- multi joint pain without joint swelling or redness
- headaches of a new type, pattern, or severity
- un-refreshing sleep
- malaise lasting more than 24 hours following exertion.

Another frequently used set of diagnostic criteria developed by Dr Michael Sharpe and colleagues in 1991 and used in the UK is the Oxford criteria,[4] which is similar to that of the Centre of Disease Control's definition (stated above) but differs in the number of signs and symptoms needed to confirm the diagnosis and, most significantly, will still diagnose CFS/ME in patients who are known to suffer from minor psychiatric disorders such as depression and anxiety states.

In 2003 Dr Bruce M. Carruthers and his Canadian colleagues published a new working case definition of CFS/ME.[5] It was the first set of criteria for the diagnosis of CFS/ME rather than the less specific term CFS. This clinical case definition, which is gradually being accepted around the world, states that in order to be diagnosed with CFS/ME the patient:

- must become symptomatically ill after exercise
- must have signs and symptoms other than fatigue, such as neurological, neurocognitive, neuroendocrine, immune manifestations and signs of autonomic disturbance.

The nineteenth century

Historically many terms have been given to CFS/ME type disorders and some of these may be different names for the same disorder. As early as 1871 Union Army doctor Dr J. M. Da Costa described a fatigue disorder that affected about three hundred soldiers during the American Civil War.[6] The soldiers had all been in active service for some while.

The signs and symptoms listed were as follows:

- abdominal problems, including diarrhoea and frequent indigestion
- palpitations usually induced by exertion
- chest pain
- shortness of breath, again aggravated by exertion
- rapid pulse
- headache and dizziness
- disturbed sleep
- excessive perspiration

Dr Da Costa noted that when the soldiers' signs and symptoms had eased, and after they had returned to duty, their performance on the battlefield was of a low standard and that they were unable to keep up with their healthy comrades. Dr Da Costa suggested that the cause of the problem was due to physical over-exertion and physical stress of the body, leading to an 'irritation of the heart'. He proposed that the condition was sustained due to an imbalance in the nerve supply to the heart, which includes sympathetic nerves. It became known as Da Costa's Syndrome, also called Irritable Heart Disease. Clinical scientist and cardiologist Sir Thomas Lewis

(1881–1945), the pioneer of the electrocardiograph, wrote a paper in 1920 noting similar cases during the First World War, which he labelled 'Effort Syndrome', also known as Neurocirculatory Asthenia. Lewis concluded that an infection was at the root of the problem.[7]

The twentieth century

Since Lewis, a number of physicians, neurologists, cardiologists and others have searched for the cause, constantly redefining this mysterious disorder. An outbreak was identified by physician Dr Melvyn Ramsay in 1955 at London's Royal Free Hospital.[1] After many doctors, nurses and patients were struck by a mysterious virus, there was one group that did not recover but continued to suffer with lethargy and a range of signs and symptoms now known to be associated with CFS/ME. The group you would expect to be most severely affected by a virus would obviously be the patients, but the sufferers of what came to be called myalgic encephalomyelitis or Royal Free disease were mostly nurses. In the 1950s nurses often had to lift heavy loads and were in a very demanding job, physically as well as mentally, placing significant strain on the spine. This is true of many CFS/ME sufferers, which, as will be explained later in the book, is no coincidence.

Eminent psychiatrists have pointed to a possible psychological source of the disease.[8] From the label Yuppie Flu of the 1980s to the dismissive attitudes of some practitioners, many patients feel isolated and depressed as a result of ignorance. The inability of most of the health care profession to legitimise this illness has been shown to aggravate psychiatric morbidity in sufferers. Sufferers have been labelled as unmotivated and school or work-phobic, although many of my patients are well motivated, high achieving type 'A' personalities.[9]

The twenty-first century

Research findings continue to lay the blame for CFS/ME on the patient's inability to cope with daily problems, fear of physical activity,[10] or altered perception of illness[11] or worse, on parental attitude such as maternal overprotection in childhood.[12] It remains a condition that attracts controversy since many of the signs and symptoms are non-specific and are common to many other illnesses, including psychiatric disorders. Depression, which is a common feature of the disease, has been viewed as a sickness behaviour seen in many chronic illnesses. CFS/ME continues to be an enigma that confounds medical research. Apart from the strain of suffering from a severely debilitating illness, much emotional stress emerges from the refusal of others to accept the validity of the illness, leading to strained relationships at home, work and school and with members of the social services and medical profession.

The patient profile

CFS/ME sufferers tend to be highly motivated individuals who were very active before the illness struck them down. They find it highly depressing being inactive. The depressed feelings and attitude of CFS/ME patients are commonly mistaken for clinical depression. Clinically depressed patients feel better when involved in increased activity, which unfortunately aggravates the symptoms of CFS/ME. CFS/ME patients feel miserable, not due to a psychiatric disorder, but from profound frustration.

The cost of CFS/ME

The UK's government's independent working group's report into chronic fatigue syndrome/myalgic encephalomyelitis in January 2002[2] estimated that a general practice with 10,000 patients was likely to have between thirty and forty CFS/ME sufferers. The prognosis for this complex disorder is recognised as very variable. The economic impact on individuals in the form of informal care and lost employment can be devastating. Statistical analysis carried out in 2003 by the Survey and Statistical Research Centre at the UK's Sheffield Hallam University revealed that CFS/ME annually costs the UK government around £3.5 billion in benefit payments, caring and loss of taxation.[13]

The rest of the world does not fare any better. An American study in 2004, by Cynthia Bierl and colleagues at the National Center for Infectious Diseases in Atlanta, found that 2.2 million American adults between the ages of 18 and 69 years suffer from CFS-like illness.[14] On a global scale the impact of CFS/ME on society in both human and economic terms is of great magnitude.

Research into CFS/ME

Although many relatively small research projects have been carried out, financed mainly by private charitable trusts, pharmaceutical firms, the main sponsors of medical research, have tended to shy away from financing any major studies investigating CFS/ME. As demonstrated from present socio-economic research, there is clearly no evidence to justify this lack of interest compared with the research funding for other global diseases such as AIDS.[15]

Some breakthroughs have been made which may mean objective clinical tests may become available to assess the severity of CFS/ME – such as a test called the head-up tilt test, using the haemodynamic instability score, which measures the change of flow and pressure of blood when the patient is placed on a tilt table, turning them upside down and then upright. In CFS/ME patients blood pressure takes longer to increase when changing from horizontal to upright and thus many feel initially faint. This phenomenon, known as neuro-mediated hypotension, is I believe due to disturbed sympathetic nerve activity, which then fails to monitor changes of position and make the correct adjustment in the cardiovascular system.[16] Yet still no universally accepted investigative tests for this condition have been validated in scientific studies. From the diagnostic viewpoint, there has been little movement in classifying the disease in over a decade, although the recent Canadian initiative to standardise the diagnostic criteria may help.[5]

The symptoms of CFS/ME typically become apparent following a common viral infection, although many other causative factors have been suggested:

- **vaccinations** against cholera, tetanus, typhoid and influenza have been associated with the onset of CFS/ME.[17]
- **organophosphate pesticides** have been suggested as an aetiological factor as have other environmental toxins.[18–21]
- patients with CFS/ME have been shown to have greater **chemical sensitivity** than healthy controls.[22,23,24]
- It has been observed that the psychological disturbances in CFS/ME occur secondary to, or share a common pathophysiology with immunological dysfunction.[25]

Important research[26] is investigating common viral gene expressions found in CFS/ME, which will help with earlier diagnosis, and perhaps some patients identified with the viral signature will soon have a treatment to help rid their body of the offending microbe. However, in many cases there appears to be no apparent cause triggering the condition.[27] Diagnosis of CFS/ME can be made only after all other medical and psychiatric causes of chronic fatiguing illnesses have been excluded.

Red blood cell structure has been studied in various diseases and findings have shown that the most common aberrant shape of a red blood cell in CFS/ME patients is a flattened disc with up to 80% of cells having this abnormal shape.[28,29] This alteration may lead to loss of fluidity and flexibility of the cell wall resulting in reduced access of these cells to the deep capillary beds, thus reducing oxygen supply to tissues and exacerbating any fatigue. Decreased concentrations of essential fatty acids in red cell membranes of CFS/ME patients were thought to be causing the malformation of the red blood cells. In fact, research at London's Hammersmith Hospital in 2003 by Professor Basant Puri has revealed a deficiency in fatty acids in CFS/ME sufferers, which are important for the healthy maintenance of all cell membranes.[30] Puri and his colleagues discovered that a combination of an omega-3 fatty acid, eicosapentaenoic acid (EPA), together with unprocessed and unrefined virgin evening primrose oil, was the best combination to restore health. However, another fatty acid, docosahexaenoic acid (DHA), when taken as a supplement, inhibits the function of EPA and thus does not help the condition and should be avoided.

A considerable body of evidence now indicates that the central nervous system is profoundly involved in the process leading to CFS/ME. Many research studies are now focusing on the high levels of toxicity found in CFS/ME patients, caused by organic solvents and heavy metals – such as mercury – which affect nerve transmission.[31–34]

The case of Miss F

Age: 18 years
Occupation: school student
Marital status: single

For three months before the start of my treatment, Miss F had been spending all day in bed. She had fallen ill suddenly in early spring, during the build-up to her Advanced Level exams. She was a grade A student who was expected to achieve just reward for the hard work and effort she had put into many years of study. Instead, she could hardly move out of her bedroom. She could not concentrate or read any book, never mind the school textbooks. Besides severe fatigue, she suffered from pain in the shoulders, arms and legs, headaches and dizziness.

She had already been diagnosed as suffering from ME by a specialist following a battery of exhaustive blood tests at her GP's practice and hospital. He had advised her to live as restful and healthy an existence as possible, and the disease would eventually burn itself out.

Her mother and father heard about the results that I was achieving with CFS/ME cases, and brought her to me for a consultation. She was virtually carried in by her parents who seemed to be desperate and looked as though they had little hope in an osteopath being able to help. Clearly her condition was very serious. On examination her spine had a badly developed curvature in the mid thoracic region, exacerbated by years of study bent over books and computers, with the upper section quite flattened. She had all the specific tender points with much lymphatic congestion in her chest and neck. Her cranial rhythm was very sluggish and hardly palpable.

Once I had examined her, I found the mechanical problems common to all my CFS/ME patients. Miss F's parents were surprised by my enthusiasm in treating their daughter, and that I was so positive that I could help her.

With an intensive course of treatment of weekly sessions over the next few months involving articulation and soft tissue massage to improve the spinal mechanics and lymph drainage and reduce muscular tone the same girl, by the end of the summer, had not only restarted her A-level course work but gained three As in her exams. She then went on to study English at university for three more years and gained a first class honours degree. After a successful career as a PA for a leading actress and film director, she is now happily married with a young baby and, most important, perfectly healthy.

Chapter 3

The role of the sympathetic nervous system in disease

It is a capital mistake to theorise before one has data.

Sir Arthur Conan Doyle 1859–1930

Many terms have been given to CFS/ME type disorders, as we saw in the previous chapter, and these may be different names for the same disease. In 1871 Dr J. M. Da Costa wrote about Da Costa's syndrome in the *American Journal of Medical Science*.[1] In this paper he suggested that the cause of the problem was physical over-exertion and stress of the body, leading to an irritation of the heart. He proposed that the condition was sustained due to an imbalance in the nerve supply to the heart. This is the earliest reference that I have discovered, to date, of a doctor proposing a similar theory to my own.

The nervous systems

The autonomic nervous system controls the automatic functions of the body. It is divided into two distinct parts: the sympathetic and parasympathetic. One of the main functions of the sympathetic nerves is the control of the walls of arteries, which supply blood to most parts of the body. (The nerve supply or 'innervation' of the heart Da Costa referred to is predominantly part of the sympathetic nervous system, with the parasympathetic vagus nerve aiding the heartbeat.) It is interesting to note that when the sympathetic nerves supplying the heart are over-active, the heart rate can increase to over 200 beats a minute, whereas the average normal adult heart rate is 50–100 beats a minute.

Da Costa's syndrome was known as 'Irritable Heart' and was also recognised in the Crimean War (1853–1856). Cardiologist, Sir Thomas Lewis noted similar cases during the First World War (1914–18), which he labelled 'Effort Syndrome'. Lewis concluded that an infection was at the root of the problem and coined the term 'Neurocirculatory Asthenia'.

Following Lewis, many physicians, neurologists, cardiologists and other scientists have searched for the cause, and, in the process, constantly redefined this mysterious disorder. From 1918, eminent psychiatrists have pointed to a possible psychological source of the disease.

The primary machinery of life

It is something of a coincidence that as well as Dr Da Costa, another physician practising during the American Civil War has been a major influence on my theories. Dr Andrew Taylor Still, shortly after serving in the Union Army, founded the mechanical treatment of the body that he termed osteopathy.

The concept of the primary machinery of the body being the neuromuscular-skeletal system, with the internal organs being secondary and supportive, is a fundamental principle of osteopathic philosophy. The role of the sympathetic nervous system is to co-ordinate this function of the viscera, via messages and impulses from the muscular skeletal system, thus allowing the healthy existence of the whole body.

When one observes a fellow human, it is the make-up of the person that is apparent – their build, and shape and how they utilise their structural assets. In everyday existence, it is the muscles, tendons, ligaments, joints, skin and bones, together with the nerves supplying these structures (the somatic nerves) that form the 'Primary Machinery of Life' as it was described by one of the past luminaries of the osteopathic world, physiologist Irvin M. Korr (1909–2004) in his studies on the autonomic nervous system.[2–6]

The sympathetic nervous system has its entire origin within the spinal cord. Along with the other part of the autonomic system, the parasympathetic nerves, as well as the hormones of the endocrine system, it is responsible for tuning visceral, circulatory and metabolic activity to muscular demand. The overall control centre of the autonomic nerves lies in the brain. However, the performance of the sympathetic system can be greatly affected by mechanical and postural strain to the mid section of the spine, from the first thoracic vertebra to the second lumbar segment.

How the sympathetic nervous system responds

Rapid adjustments in accordance with levels of exertion and posture are orchestrated largely by the sympathetic nerves. The parasympathetic system makes long-term adjustments maintaining and replenishing stores of nutrients and fuel, which have been utilised under the direction of the sympathetic system. In other words, both sections of the autonomic nervous system work in conjunction with each other. From this viewpoint, illness results from the inconsistency between demands of the neuromuscular-skeletal system (the primary machinery) and the ability to maintain adequate provision for the normal functioning of all of the body's systems. Thus a patient requires rest when ill, reducing demands until this disparity is corrected.

Traditional medicine places an emphasis on the demands made by the internal organs; however, by virtue of their mass and their rapidly changing metabolic rate, the muscles are the main consumers of the body's energy supply.

Four possible causes of disease within the body exist:

1. Damage to the neuromuscular-skeletal system due to trauma, postural problems or over-use.
2. Visceral disorders (disorders of the internal organs) due to physical or operational defects in one or more of these organs.
3. Emotional or psychosomatic disorders.
4. Communicative disorders, which occur when there is impaired communication between the musculoskeletal system and the internal organs. This happens when either the nervous or vascular channels are either incomplete or interrupted.

CFS/ME falls into this fourth category.

Organisation of the automatic nervous system

Different nerve fibres join each other at points known as synapses. In the autonomic nervous system, a large number of nerves join each other in separate bundles of synapses. These bundles of nervous tissue are situated throughout the body and are each known as a ganglion. The nerves between the spinal cord and the ganglia are known as preganglionic, and the nerves between the ganglia and the target organ are called postganglionic fibres. One preganglionic fibre may synapse with many postganglionic nerves, thus increasing the overall area in the body affected by one impulse from the spine.

The sympathetic ganglia mostly lie at the side of the middle section of the spinal cord in two parallel chains (the sympathetic trunks). There are other sympathetic ganglia that lie in front of the main artery in the abdomen, the aorta. Some form large bundles of nerve fibres, each known as a plexus, which create sensitive areas, for example, the solar plexus.

The parasympathetic ganglia are mainly situated in the organ supplied. Their postganglionic fibres innervate all the internal organs and the eye. The uppermost fibres in the head supply the lachrymal glands of the eye, which produce tears, and the salivary glands. A major parasympathetic nerve from the head is the vagus, which supplies the organs of the neck, thorax, pelvis and genitalia.

The sympathetic postganglionic fibres supply all the organs innervated by the parasympathetic nerves, although the distribution to different parts of the organ may vary. The blood supply to the body is almost entirely under the control of the sympathetic nervous system, except the vasculature of the pelvic organs and genitalia, which is under parasympathetic regulation.

The sympathetic influence over the arterial pressure and the peripheral blood resistance affects the cardiac output and many other metabolic processes. The parasympathetic vagus nerve modifies the rhythm of the heart, but the sympathetic nerves regulate the entire cardiovascular system, in accordance with what is going on in the body as a whole.

In summary, the sympathetic nervous system differs from the parasympathetic in these key ways:

1. The parasympathetic nerve supply is almost entirely visceral, exerting most of its control over the internal organs. The sympathetic nerves, however, regulate functioning of the skin, bones, ligaments, tendons and parts of the somatic nervous system, plus the skeletal muscle as well as the organs.
2. The parasympathetic nerves are more specific, with individual nerves supplying a specific target organ. The sympathetic effects are more widespread due to a fanning out of the nerves to all the tissues.
3. The parasympathetic nerves control blood supply only to the genitalia. The sympathetic nerves control the circulation throughout the rest of the body. This is why impotence is rarely complained of in CFS/ME, as it is not caused by sympathetic disturbance. Sexual intercourse is usually a problem due to lack of libido or just plain exhaustion
4. The parasympathetic system is not directly affected by the requirements of the body, but the sympathetic nerves are influenced and controlled by the demands of the other bodily systems.

Control of blood flow by the sympathetic nervous system

Research in the 1930s by Dale, Feldberg and Gaddum[7,8] revealed that the transport of nerve impulses across synapses involved the release of chemicals known as neurotransmitters. There are two types of neurotransmitters involved in the autonomic control of the viscera:

1. the cholinergic neurotransmitters – which use the chemical acetylcholine;
2. the adrenergic neurotransmitters – which use noradrenaline (or 'norephinephrine' in the US).

One of the main transmitter substances in the sympathetic nervous system is noradrenaline. This is formed in a small organ in the brain stem known as the locus coruleus, which is under the direct influence of the hypothalamus.

Further investigation has found that the hormone adrenaline (or 'epinephrine') acts on two receptors at the target organ. These receptors are called alpha- and beta-receptors. When an alpha-receptor is stimulated, it causes constriction of the blood vessels. Vasodilation (dilation of the blood vessels) occurs if the beta-receptors are excited. Thus adrenaline can produce an increase and decrease of blood flow. The neurotransmitter noradrenaline, on the other hand, predominantly acts on alpha-receptors, leading to vasoconstriction.

More research has discovered a further division of the receptors of the neurochemical transmitters, alpha 1 and alpha 2 plus beta 1 and beta 2. The transfer of messages to the four receptors is blocked by different chemical antagonists, e.g. the antagonist drug prazosin blocks only alpha 1 receptors. Stimulation of the alpha 1 receptors leads to constriction of the blood vessels; thus the prazosin, by blocking this effect, aids vasodilation thus reducing the overall blood pressure. This is because the larger the diameter of the vessels the less the resistance against the flow of blood. This selectivity makes the alpha-adrenergic blocker, prazosin, useful in treating hypertension (high blood pressure).

The sympathetic nervous system maintains an important function in regulating the body's inner environment. This process, known as homeostasis, is clearly demonstrated when there is a break of the spinal cord above the first thoracic vertebra following a major trauma. The lesion of the cord at this level would cut off the whole thoracic-lumbar sympathetic outflow from higher control. After such an accident, tilting the patient from supine (lying down) to an upright position would lead to:

- decrease in blood pressure
- increase in the rate of the pulse
- loss of consciousness.

These effects occur since there is no compensatory control of the blood vessels to adjust to the change of position. The skin blood vessels do not adapt to any change of body temperature, so there is no vasodilation or sweating. If cold there is no shivering of the muscles controlled by nerves below the spinal lesion. It is important to note that the lower the damage to the cord, the smaller the disturbance of the autonomic control.

Sympathetic fibres reach the blood vessels via two distinct paths:

1. directly, from the sympathetic chain to the plexuses around the aorta controlling the vessels in the abdomen, thorax, skull and upper parts of the arms and legs;
2. indirectly via peripheral nerves to the forearms, hands, lower legs and feet. Surgeons often help circulatory problems by an operation known as a sympathectomy. The results of this form of surgery include widespread and lasting dilation of the arterial supply in the limbs, especially in the skin.

If the signs and symptoms of CFS/ME are due to a dysfunction of the sympathetic nervous system, a sympathectomy is obviously not the desired treatment; although the peripheral circulation may improve, cutting off the sympathetic control would have unwanted side-effects. This is also the case with beta-blockers, which are regularly prescribed for cardiovascular signs and symptoms such as palpitations or high blood pressure. In most CFS/ME patients beta-blockers will exacerbate the fatigue and should be avoided if possible.

Pain, numbness and muscle spasm in CFS/ME

An intimate relationship exists between part of the somatic nervous system and the sympathetic nerves. The somatic motor nerves, which stimulate skeletal muscle contraction, contain fibres that lie alongside the fibres of the sympathetic nerves as they leave the spinal cord. The sympathetic fibres connect with the motor nerves as they travel down to the tissues being supplied.

The sympathetic sensory nerves are excited by painful states in the internal organs. The reduction of blood flow when there is a spasm in the organ leads to a chemical irritation stimulating the preganglionic sympathetic nerves in the spinal cord. This leads to physiological changes within the target organs, e.g. dilation of blood vessels resulting in increased circulation. The neighbouring motor-neurones are excited, prompting a sustained muscular contraction, for example, muscle spasm and pain in the right shoulder in cases of gall bladder inflammation. This is a classic example of what is known as referred pain, in which pain is felt at one site of the body although its cause lies within another part of the body.

A case of referred pain

An elderly man visited my practice, complaining of an ache in the right shoulder. He informed me that all he needed was a 'good rub' on the offending joint. I took his full medical history and carried out an examination, as is usual practice, before treatment. As I took his medical history, it emerged that the shoulder pain worsened after eating fatty or fried foods. When I examined the region of the gall bladder in the upper right section of the abdomen, underneath the ninth rib, I noted that pressure caused the patient severe pain. This positive test, known as Murphy's sign, confirmed my suspicions, and I promptly sent the patient to hospital. The following day he had successful surgery on his gall bladder, to remove a large stone. The shoulder pain disappeared soon after his operation. This case demonstrates how the sympathetic nerves' connections with the somatic nervous system co-exist.

The reason for this referred pain is complex but is due to mainly to the following mechanisms.

Sympathetic nerves are small fibre nerves. In other words their cross section is much smaller than the somatic nerves that control movement and sensation in our body. To protect the sympathetic nerves from damage they lie alongside the thicker somatic nerves as they leave and travel back to the spinal cord. Sympathetic nerves, due to their close proximity to sensory somatic nerves, are equally sensitive to stimuli such as pain as a result of 'cross talk' of nerve impulses travelling from one nerve to the adjacent one (Gasser, 1955).

The connection between pain receptors and sympathetic nerves has been observed in many disease states (Janig, 1988).

Influence has also been noted via activity of the sympathetic nerves stimulating pain-inducing chemicals to be released and specialised nerve receptors to fire off impulses that eventually lead to pain.

Transmitters released at peripheral endings of nerves produce localised increased blood flow. Furthermore, they may have effects on the regional immune cells leading to what is known as 'neurogenic inflammation', with eventual stimulation sensory fibres causing pain (Mense, 2004). This may also explain many of the more severe musculo-skeletal and sensory symptoms affecting the patient with CFS/ME.

Stimulation of the sympathetic nervous system

If the sympathetic system is over-stimulated, it causes[9,10] the following effects:

1. The force of muscle contraction is increased and there appears to be a delay in the onset of fatigue in over-stimulated muscles.
2. There is an increase in excitability of sensory mechanisms. By cross-over of nerve impulses from sympathetic nerves to sensory nerves this may present as increase in pain and/or enhanced sensitivity to light, sound and smells.
3. The bone marrow, which is very rich in sympathetic nerve supply, is stimulated to fight any disease.
4. The endocrine system, which is under the influence of the sympathetic nerves, is stimulated to release hormones from glands such as the thyroid, adrenals and pancreas.

It therefore follows that if there is impairment in sympathetic control, the opposite effects may occur, thus reducing muscle contraction, increasing fatigue, reducing sensation and lowering resistance to disease.

Sympathetic stimulation only modifies the inherent physiology rather than introducing new qualities, so that each tissue responds in its own particular way. This is why CFS/ME can affect different patients in various ways. Some sympathetic paths may be functioning correctly, others may be overactive, while in other cases they may be severely blocked. The common factor is that with any form of CFS/ME there is a general disorder, or dysfunction of the sympathetic nervous system as a whole, causing widespread signs and symptoms of ill health within the body. Some of the signs and symptoms are due to an over-activity of the sympathetic nerves, other effects relate to a reduction of sympathetic activity.

Sir Thomas Lewis[11] observed in the 1930s that the patients with 'Effort Syndrome' displayed a characteristic drooping posture, which he attributed to the fatigue and depression they suffered. The concept that the bad posture might be causing the disorder in the first place evaded him. The mechanical strain that a kyphotic, or bowed, upper spine places upon the sympathetic nervous system is immense and, over a period of time, can directly lead to the patient developing CFS/ME.

How viruses affect nerves

As mentioned at the beginning of the chapter, Lewis surmised that the disorder was due to an infection. An infection is defined as the invasion of tissues by living micro-organisms. Disease is produced by their subsequent multiplication. Bacteria and viruses are the most common type of pathogenic (disease producing) organisms in man. It is a widely held belief that a virus is the underlying cause of CFS/ME. Many practitioners still refer to the illness as Post-Viral Fatigue syndrome. They believe a virus was initially present in the body and has caused long term damage to the body or remains dormant waiting to inflict damage at a later date. A virus would be the most plausible explanation when dealing with certain recorded outbreaks of CFS/ME, where the incidence has almost reached epidemic proportions, for example, at the Royal Free Hospital, London in 1955.[12]

A virus is the smallest micro-organism known, measuring only nanometers in length (one meter = one billion nanometres). Viruses sometimes are known to attack specific parts of the nervous system. A well-known viral infection, shingles, affects sensory nerves due to the virus *Herpes zoster*. With shingles there is an initial infection by the virus, usually in childhood, causing chicken pox. The child recovers but the virus lies dormant for many years in the root of a sensory nerve as it leaves the spinal cord. Eventually, the virus may reactivate in the form of shingles. This is an example of a latent virus infection.

A well-known viral infection that involves the central nervous system is polio (polio myelitis). The infection occurs after the virus has entered the body via the mouth (in food or drink). The virus then attacks specific cells in part of the spinal cord. There is a tendency for the polio virus to affect the lumbar region, in the lower section of the cord, more than the dorsal or cervical areas.

Another serious infection that affects the nervous system is Creutzfeldt-Jakob disease (CJD), a rare and ultimately fatal progressive degenerative brain disease caused by the build up in the brain of an abnormal form of the naturally occurring 'prion' protein. Prions are abnormal forms of protein that are extremely difficult to destroy. Their presence in the brain causes spongiform encephalopathy, so-called because areas where cells have died take on a sponge-like appearance when viewed under the microscope. There is a type of CJD known as variant CJD which is thought to be caused by bovine spongiform encephalopathy (BSE), a form of prion disease affecting cattle. Prion diseases have been found in several other animal species, including sheep (scrapie), deer and cats. The consumption of infected beef products appears to have led to the development of BSE in humans.

This demonstrates that viruses and other infectious agents are capable of targeting precise regions of the spine, and concentrating their effect on particular nerve cells. This may be precisely what occurs with CFS/ME, with the unknown virus attacking the thoracic and upper lumbar areas, acting on the sympathetic nerves or ganglia.

In the 1980s epidemics in a number of American towns broke out, where blood tests showed that the patients had been infected with the Epstein-Barr virus,[13,14,15] the herpes virus that causes glandular fever. However, the signs and symptoms were different from glandular fever, and the patients seemed to be suffering from different viruses at the same time. This led many U.S. doctors to refer to the disease as Chronic Epstein-Barr Virus Syndrome.

Researchers have concentrated on other viruses, namely polio, Coxsackie's and a recently discovered Herpes HHV-6,[16,17] but none has shown up exclusively in every patient with CFS/ME. I believe the long-term irritation of the brain, hormonal system, and ultimately the sympathetic nervous system leads to a disorder in the normal function of the blood circulation, and visceral activity, which directly affects the immune system. This results in the body as a whole being susceptible to viral infections of more than one type.

Infectious diseases usually focus on weak areas in the victim's body. If a virus is to blame for CFS/ME, then a long-term irritation of the sympathetic nerves could lead to a weakness in that system, which may render it prone to a viral infection.

Genetics research

This chronic sympathetic irritation may stem from a postural problem of the thoracic and upper lumbar spine. Although bad posture may be brought about by unhealthy habits, for example, slouching in soft easy chairs, the shape of the back may be determined by genetic factors. As in all areas of medicine, genetic research has a major role to play in improving our future understanding of aetiological mechanisms that may pre-dispose patients to CFS/ME. Variant genotypes associated with muscle metabolism and physical endurance have been discovered in Gulf War veterans that would make them much more likely to develop CFS/ME.[18] Clinically one can see a genetic pattern in the family history data where there is more than one family member with CFS/ME. There have been cases of occurrences of the disorder in three generations.

Just as the colour of one's eyes and hair are hereditary, so can stiffness and curvature of the spine, and developmental problems in the cranium run in families. Structural anomalies of cranial bones have been linked to genetic mutation, as have spinal deformities. [19,20] A virus may strike at those in the unfortunate family who possess the same mechanical problem of the spine. This could be why there are reported cases of a few members of the same household suffering from CFS/ME.

Pre-viral or post-viral?

My hypothesis does not rule out the possibility of viruses being involved in the pathology of CFS/ME. However, I believe that the condition is pre-viral rather than post-viral. I believe that the sympathetic nervous system's dysfunction leads to an impairment of the body's immune system. This in turn results in the entire body becoming susceptible to viral infections of more than one type. This explains why research into viral causes has been going on for some years, with many different viruses being suspected of playing a role in the establishment of the disease, but with no conclusive findings.

Just as Sir Thomas Lewis wrongly concluded that the poor posture he saw in his patients was a result of the fatigued and depressed state of the body and not part of the cause, so I believe that viral infectious diseases occur as a result of CFS/ME and are not the creators of the disease. This, I believe, is why, in the very early stages of the disorder, only a mechanical and postural-based examination can detect the development of this disorder before the sympathetic nervous system breaks down. In other words, CFS/ME is preventable if treated and managed properly in the early stages.

If disturbance of the sympathetic nervous system is allowed to take place, the ultimate result is the manifestation of the many signs and symptoms and complications that we now associate with CFS/ME.

The case of Mr C

Age: 34 years
Occupation: Managing director of department store
Marital status: Married with three young children.

Mr C initially complained of tightness in both shoulders and upper back. He also suffered from general fatigue and aching in his arms and legs, with occasional pins and needles in his hands and feet, and he experienced frequent chest pains.

(I have found that pain in the chest is a frequent symptom in CFS/ME. Unfortunately, this tenderness may add to the patient's anxiety. Many sufferers, especially men, believe that their heart is about to pack up, while many women suspect the onset of breast cancer. The likely cause of chest pain in CFS/ME sufferers is a combination of the overall fatigue affecting the

pectoral muscles, together with the postural strain exerted on the rib cage, plus lymphatic drainage problems.)

Mr C felt a steadily increasing loss of strength in both his arms and legs, and was convinced his muscle bulk was wasting. He was also aware of a heightened sensitivity in the joints of his limbs, especially in his elbows.

Besides the sympathetic disturbances, the symptoms suggested the existence of an irritation of the somatic, or sensory, nerves. In most cases of CFS/ME, there is no muscle wastage except from lack of use. Both increased and decreased sensitivity to feeling touch, sound and light are common symptoms in CFS/ME.

His doctor had diagnosed Mr C with anxiety, but Mr C had declined any form of sedative. When he first arrived at my practice, he presented with a restricted upper dorsal spine, and an increase of muscle tone in the upper back and shoulders. I started manipulative treatment and prescribed mobility exercises.

Mr C did not stop working, although, at weekends when he was resting, he noticed that his symptoms improved. After an initial, intensive course of therapy, comprising fourteen 30-minute treatment sessions, Mr C felt far less anxious. His back and shoulders were noticeably more relaxed, but the tension and hypersensitivity in his arms were still present. Detailed measurement of the muscle bulk in his arms revealed an increase in the muscle size since treatment commenced.

Although there was a definite overall improvement in the symptoms, his body was not being given the chance to recover fully. Work was to blame for prolonging his discomfort. I advised him to take a well-deserved rest. He eventually took a two-week break in the sun with his family.

Mr C returned every three months for check-ups and gradually looked and felt much improved and, eventually, was discharged without any sedatives being necessary.

Chapter 4

The causes of CFS/ME

> The person who strays away from the source is unroofed and is like dust blown about by the wind.
>
> *Molefi Kete Asante (1942–) US educator*

Considerable controversy surrounds the cause or causes of CFS/ME. This chapter looks at the following possibilities:

- Immunological
- Inflammatory
- Viral
- Hormonal imbalance
- Depression
- Allergy and sensitivity
- Oxidative stress.

Immunological disorder

Many people believe that CFS/ME is an immune disorder[1–4] that enables viruses, which are normally controlled within the body, to go rampant and start to attack healthy body tissue in a similar way to AIDS, but without fatal consequences.

The immune system utilises helper T-cells, also known as thymus-dependent lymphocytes, which are cells that circulate through the blood and lymph nodes for many years waiting to attack foreign material that has invaded the body. They are produced in the thymus gland that lies in the upper part of the chest. The thymus gland is a vital part of the immune system.

The immune system produces chemicals as markers that enable the killer cells to blitz the bugs. These chemicals, known as cytokines, produce nasty side-effects such as sickness and lethargy. Patients with CFS/ME initially have an overactive immune system producing far too many T-cells. Certain enzymes, which help drive the immune reaction such as RNaseL, have been shown to be overactive.[5–7] This leads to an interesting phenomenon experienced by most CFS/ME patients, at least in the early stages of the disease. Their families and friends may suffer from the occasional cold and bout of flu but CFS/ME patients will just feel groggy and weak with a worsening of their usual symptoms but without full-blown cold or flu symptoms. This is because the viruses in their upper respiratory tract are already being blasted by far too many T-cells, and, consequently, the usual viral symptoms, which are due to the normal immune response, do not occur.

After a while this situation may reverse and the immune system may become severely depressed, with the patient suffering from constant recurrent infections.

Many symptoms associated with CFS/ME, such as enlarged lymph glands, fever, gut symptoms, recurrent respiratory infections and pharyngitis, appear to indicate an immunological disorder. Indeed, the onset of the disease often appears to follow a viral infection. The body provides two basic forms of immune response: humoral and cellular (cell-mediated). Both forms are co-ordinated by the cells of the immune system and their mediators.

Humoral immunity

Humoral immunity is the major defence mechanism against bacterial infections and utilises circulating antibodies that are produced by specialised cells, B-cells, supported by other cells called T-helper/inducer cells. After recognising foreign material B-cells multiply rapidly and produce antibodies comprised of large immunoglobulins. These protein molecules are produced in large numbers and are usually specific to the infective or foreign agent. The antibodies form complexes with the foreign material and these complexes are then destroyed by other cells, such as macrophages.

Cellular (cell-mediated) immunity

Cellular immunity involves a variety of T-cells that are responsible for protection against viruses, cancers, and some disease-causing bacteria such as tuberculosis.

T-helper (Th) cells assist B-cells in mounting a humoral response and cytotoxic T lymphocytes (Tc) can actively destroy abnormal cells in disease and malignancies. A further group of cells are natural killer (NK) cells, which play an important part in counteracting viral infections and cancer.

The complex interactions between all the B- and T-cells require cytokines (mentioned above), which are large protein signalling molecules. There are many types of cytokines, which are subdivided into smaller groups (e.g. interleukins and interferons). During an infection both T- and B-cells multiply rapidly, with cell numbers returning to normal levels after the antigen has been defeated. However, some memory cells remain so that a second infection is more rapidly combated. Some research findings[8,9] have demonstrated a cytokine involvement in the pathophysiological mechanisms found in CFS/ME.

The inflammatory response

Inflammation is a complex response to localised injury and trauma and, although it is usually an acute response, there are a number of well-known chronic inflammatory diseases such as rheumatoid arthritis and sinusitis. The inflammatory response involves cytokines together with other classes of inflammatory modulators such as certain prostaglandins.

The recent controversy about the part of the MMR (measles, mumps and rubella) vaccine being associated with the development of autism involved the identification of grossly inflamed tissue in the lower part of the small intestine.[10] Inflammation of this part of the gut is common among CFS/ME patients and many have been diagnosed with irritable bowel syndrome, inflammatory bowel disease, and Crohn's disease. Allergic reactions to food containing gluten are common. The best known of these is coeliac disease in which the structure of the small bowel is destroyed, with a flattening of the deeply folded villi of the gut wall, and diminished capacity properly to absorb many key nutrients from food. Generally, CFS/ME patients do not test positive for coeliac disease but many become sensitive to chemicals and foodstuffs, especially gluten.

When digestion is impaired, the larger peptide fragments in food are not broken down. Among these are opioid peptides derived from two principal sources, casein in milk (the casomorphins) and gliadin in gluten (the gliadomorphins), which occur in wheat and other cereal crops such as rye and barley. Opioids are peptides that have been found to possess morphine-like activity and are known to be naturally occurring in important transmitter molecules, particularly in the gut, brain and immune system.

When the gut wall has increased permeability, these opioid peptides, which would normally be excluded, are absorbed and act both locally in the gut and in other organs, particularly the brain. The same factors that render the gut permeable appear to increase the permeability of the blood-brain barrier and allow access of these compounds to the brain.

Depending on the concentration of opioids in the gut, as well as permeability of the gut and blood-brain barrier, the overall level of these compounds in the bloodstream and the brain may vary and give rise to variable expressions of symptoms and dysfunction. Opioids play a significant part in the immune response through receptors found on cells of the immune system. Generally, they suppress the immune response and increase susceptibility to infection.

The gut and the brain communicate via messenger molecules generated by the immune response. There are receptors on brain cells for cytokines.

Sometimes the process that leads to CFS/ME may be linked to other more serious illness. A subset of disease-free breast cancer patients complained of a range of symptoms almost identical to CFS/ME sufferers, such as fatigue and loss of concentration.[11] A previous link was made between non-Hodgkin's lymphomas and CFS/ME following a 1988 epidemiological investigation into a cluster of CFS/ME sufferers in North Carolina.[12]

The symptoms and signs of CFS/ME are very similar to Addison's disease (primary adrenal insufficiency). However, corticosteroid replacement, where there are no physical signs of adrenal compromise, is clearly unwarranted, as it would further exacerbate signs and symptoms. In fact, the only physical sign of adrenal dysfunction I have observed in CFS/ME is one usually attributed to high levels of cortisol, namely striae gravida (stretch marks), which are seen in Cushing's syndrome.

Detoxification systems in the liver play a key part in the generalised stress response via their role in dealing with the metabolic products of stress. The gut has a complex immune system network controlled by an elaborate nerve supply that produces a number of neurotransmitters. Lymphocytes in the gut secrete small amounts of hormones that are thought to play a local part in regulating inflammation in the gut. It is possible that the release of hormones in the gut is influenced by stress. It is conceivable that these impairments may be a result of disrupted communications in the neuroimmune network.

The immune system has been shown to exert numerous effects on the hypothalamus and thus the autonomic nervous system. Immune activation is associated with increased firing rates of hypothalamic neurones. Activated immune cells release cytokines that are important mediators of the stress response. It is known that activated immune cells can cross the blood-brain barrier and release cytokines and other immune mediators into the central nervous system. Central and peripheral administration of cytokines affects a range of behaviours, including feeding, sleeping, drinking, levels of activity and mood, presumably by their action on receptor sites in the limbic system. Infections have an effect on the limbic system, which plays a major part in regulating memory and learning, and is directly involved in hypothalamic and autonomic function. Dysfunction of the limbic system in the brain may lead to many of the symptoms associated with CFS/ME and explain why these patients are very sensitive to both physical and psychological stress.[13] Functional changes in limbic areas have been demonstrated in CFS/ME using SPECT scans (single-photon emission computerised tomography).[14] The limbic system controls emotions and dream states and it is significant that patients with CFS/ME often complain of mood swings and weird or extremely vivid dreams, nightmares or, in some cases, hallucinations.

The viral trigger

Some viruses have been implicated as possible causal factors in CFS/ME, as noted in Chapter 3. A class of virus, known as enteroviruses – such as the Coxsackie B group – are believed to be particularly important in triggering CFS/ME.[15] Treatment approaches over recent years have focused on antiviral medications. However, most antiviral treatments have very unpleasant side effects and should be used with caution.

The antiviral drug val acyclovir has undergone vigorous tests[16] to analyse its efficacy in treating CFS/ME. Acyclovir has been successful against the Epstein-Barr virus, but double-blind trials have shown it to have no greater effect on CFS/ME than a placebo.[17] Most patients on the acyclovir drug trials reported that any improvement was short-lived and their symptoms returned soon after the treatment was completed.

Hormonal imbalance

The hypothalamus is the portion of the brain that controls and receives messages from the sympathetic nervous system. As we have seen (page 5) it becomes dysfunctional in CFS/ME. It also controls the release of the body's hormones, thus hypothalamic dysfunction in CFS/ME may affect the entire endocrine system. Therefore, one might find excesses or deficiencies in many hormonal levels in patients with the disease. Both raised[18] and reduced levels[19] of a precursor of the major sex hormones – serum dehydroepiandrosterone (DHEA-S) – secreted from the adrenal glands, have been found in CFS/ME sufferers. As with many hormones, both high and low levels of melatonin, produced by the pineal gland, have been reported in a sample of patients with CFS/ME. Melatonin levels are found to be high when daytime drowsiness and excessive sleep are reported.[20] However, when insomnia is a major symptom, supplements of melatonin usually prove to be beneficial.[21]

Insulin-like growth factor (IGF-1), the main mediator of growth hormone effects, is found to be reduced in CFS/ME sufferers. Growth hormone has been used to treat CFS/ME patients, showing a significant improvement in symptoms after six months in the experimental group compared with the control group of patients treated with a placebo.[22] However, the improvement proved short lived after medication was discontinued.

Depression

The secondary feeling of depression and anxiety in CFS/ME is different to primary depression. However, antidepressant drugs have been used for symptomatic relief in many non-psychiatric illnesses such as Parkinson's disease, multiple sclerosis and hypothyroidism. In the same way, antidepressants can sometimes reduce the signs and symptoms of CFS/ME; however, symptomatic improvement occurs at much lower doses and more rapidly than in depression. Many patients with CFS/ME who find it difficult to relax when trying to fall asleep are regularly advised to take 10 to 25 mg of amitriptyline one hour before retiring to bed. This is significantly less than the normal dose of this mild tricyclic antidepressant, which when prescribed for anxiety/depression is 150 mg a day. When the patient suffers with high anxiety a low dose of the selective serotonin re-uptake inhibitor (SSRI) type antidepressant, such as sertraline hydrochloride, has been shown to help but should be taken with caution.

Many patients with CFS/ME cannot tolerate the effects of SSRI antidepressants such as fluoxetine because they increase the amount of the neurotransmitter serotonin within the nervous system. Too much serotonin will overload the sympathetic nervous system aggravating most of the symptoms associated with CFS/ME. Thus dropout rates from studies of antidepressant therapy in CFS/ME exceed those of patients with depression.[23–24] Signs and symptoms of depression in CFS/ME may occasionally be sufficiently severe to require full dose antidepressant therapy; however, the patients in these cases may have two distinct disorders, 1. CFS/ME and 2. clinical depression. Patients are of course allowed to have more than one thing wrong with them at a time! However, mostly the symptoms of depression are secondary to suffering such a depressing disorder as CFS/ME, which I term TFUS (Thoroughly Fed Up Syndrome).

Allergy and sensitivity

As already discussed (pages 31–38) CFS/ME directly affects the immune mechanisms. Besides making the patient more susceptible to infections, it usually reduces the body's capacity to cope with allergens, leading to increased intolerance to pollen, chemicals or foods. Some CFS/ME patients, with high levels of sensitivity bordering on allergy, have been treated by Miller neutralisation. The Miller technique involves provocation of the skin followed by the administration of a neutralisation 'vaccine' of individual allergens. It acts by stimulating the body to produce higher levels of detoxification enzymes, thus helping the body cope with the allergen.[25]

Enzyme-potentiated desensitisation (EPD) is another anti-allergy treatment that has benefited many CFS/ME patients by actively adding enzymes to enhance the desensitising effect and is applied to a scratch on the skin or by intradermal injection.[26]

Oxidative stress

Oxidative stress has been acknowledged as a common feature in many disease processes, including CFS/ME. Oxidative stress may induce many of the symptoms of CFS/ME. Excessive production of the free radical nitric oxide may damage the central nervous system. In an atom small negative charged electrons spin around the central nucleus, akin to planets orbiting the sun. Some atoms have electrons on their outer rings that are shared with other atoms. A group of atoms join to form a larger molecule. A free radical is a molecule with an atom that has lost one of these shared electrons from their outer ring. This will make it highly unstable and it will damage healthy tissue by trying to obtain another electron from an adjacent molecule. Oxygen reacts with free radicals to form peroxidised radicals, which further damage healthy molecules. Oxidative stress increases free radical production leading to further cell damage and worsening toxicity. External factors, such as environmental pollutants and radiation, can lead to major free radical production. Overall nitric oxide synthesis is increased in CFS/ME and may be induced by inflammatory cytokines.[27] The neurotoxic effect is further aggravated by amplified sensitivity due to increased nitric oxide stimulation of the neurotransmitter glutamate.[28]

Antioxidants restore free radicals to healthy molecules. Antioxidants such as vitamin C have been shown to be major combatants in fighting disease ever since the 1950s when Harman[29] discovered the part played by free radicals. The rationale for vitamin C infusion in CFS/ME rests on the traditional use of megadose vitamin C infusion treatments in autoimmune disease, allergy and a range of other conditions.[30]

Multiple chemical sensitivity, together with raised nitric oxide, plus an increase in blood–brain barrier permeability and gut wall permeability, leads to a group of patients with an inability to prevent toxic overload within the central nervous system. Furthermore, this leads to an inability to cope with the toxins.

The case of the Reverend B

Age: 48 years
Occupation: Community chaplain
Marital status: Married with 6 children.

The Reverend B had initially consulted me six years previously, when he had suffered from a mechanical strain of the neck. He had collapsed two years before that but no abnormality was detected at that time by his GP. His earlier neck problem was linked to his overall poor posture, especially in the middle part of his back, the dorsal spine, which was severely kyphotic (bent forward) and showed marked spondylotic changes. (Spondylitis is the name given to arthritis of the spine.)

In August 1990 he consulted me complaining of dizziness, nausea, frequent headaches and general fatigue, which was aggravated by exertion. He also complained of pain in both his legs, which worsened after an anti-tetanus injection. He was referred by his doctor to a neurologist, who examined him thoroughly but found no abnormalities. By the time he came to my practice, he was unable to walk. A taxi ferried him between my rooms and his house and, sadly, apart from these treatment sessions he was a virtual prisoner in his own home. He was obviously incapable of working and was clearly depressed about his inability to carry out his pastoral and educational duties.

This case may appear similar to Mr C (see Chapter 3), both with an obvious mechanical strain on the dorsal spine leading to symptoms of fatigue. However, there was one major difference that led to more severe problems affecting the minister. His symptoms were caused by an arthritic condition, leading to a permanent and restrictive disorder of the spine, whereas Mr C's problem was due to bad posture adopted at home and at his shop.

Corrective exercises, together with spinal manipulation and massage, improved the spinal mechanics of the shopkeeper to bring about a total lasting cure. Unfortunately, this was not the case with the chaplain. Since his CFS/ME, in my estimation, was due to a permanent irritation of the dorsal spine, I could see no hope of a cure, until somebody found a panacea for arthritis. The best I could offer was to help relieve the symptoms.

Fifteen treatments over the first year produced encouraging signs of improvement. The dizziness became less frequent, and he found himself able to take short strolls up the street with less difficulty. Having been housebound, he was now able to lead a more normal existence. For many years after there was still some weakness, especially in his legs, but as the years have gone by he has felt less lethargic, with his headaches and dizziness occurring only very occasionally. He still continues the exercises prescribed during the early stages of treatment, which maintain as much mobility as possible in his thoracic spine.

Chapter 5

How CFS/ME is treated

> The healer of those that are broken in heart and the One Who binds up their sorrows
>
> *Book of Psalms CXLVII, verse 3*

No one can be certain of the best possible treatment for CFS/ME until the cause is established and accepted. However, the one common feature of all the treatments for CFS/ME is the removal of stress-producing factors. We know that stress is damaging the body in some way or another, whether it is through too much yeast, too little magnesium or a viral infection (see below).

A build-up of stress in the body eventually reaches a point at which the slightest overload causes a complete collapse. This is similar to a child building a tower of dominoes, one on top of another. Sooner or later, one too many will cause the whole stack to become unbalanced and collapse.

The accumulation of any stress in the body can be due to many causes, but, by treating each individual stress factor separately, rather than the problem as a whole, the pressure on the body may be reduced but will not be totally alleviated.

Current therapies used to treat CFS/ME are based on differing opinions as to the cause of the disorder. I described these possible causes in Chapter 4, including:

- Immunological factors
- Inflammation
- Viral infection
- Hormonal imbalance

- Depression
- Allergy and sensitivity
- Oxidative stress.

One has to treat all the causative factors together in order to reverse the whole process and therefore in this chapter I will consider:

- Diet in general
- Elimination and avoidance diets
- Supplements
- Immunological therapies
- Graded activity
- Exercise
- Cognitive behavioural therapy (CBT)
- Antidepressants
- Hypnosis
- My manual treatment programme.

Diet

In the wild when animals are poisoned they naturally seek out waterholes. With CFS/ME one should drink around 2 litres of fluids such as mineral or filtered water every day. This helps with detoxification, but care should be taken not to drink too much. Simple sensible dietetic practices should be followed, such as avoiding foods with too many additives, artificial flavourings and colourings and rejecting junk food whenever possible.

Elimination and avoidance diets

Many CFS/ME patients suffer from food intolerances. Diets, including low carbohydrate, gluten-free and yeast-free, have all been proposed. However, nutritionists Morris and Stare of Harvard Medical School[6] found that there is no clinical scientific evidence to substantiate claims about the efficacy of various dietary approaches in the treatment of CFS/ME.

Infection with the yeast *Candida albicans* has been cited as a cause of CFS/ME (see page 47) and can cause a chronic candidiasis hypersensitivity syndrome (CCHS). In 1989 Renfro and co-workers[1] noted that the 'yeast connection' is frequently a self-diagnosed condition on the basis of having typical symptoms and a history of frequent yeast infections and multiple courses of antibiotics. Diets are available to eliminate the yeast *Candida albicans* by avoiding the foods on which Candida thrives, for example, sugar. Low sugar diets are recommended as a means of combating Candida overgrowth, as yeast requires sugar for metabolism. However, there is little scientific evidence that such regimes do control Candida overgrowth. In addition, these diets are nutritionally unbalanced and, if followed for longer than two to three months, could result in long-term nutritional deficiencies, which would impair a return to full health.

The usual dietetic advice that works best for most CFS/ME sufferers is that the patient should eat healthy, regular meals, and vary the types of food. Eating the same food types again and again may stimulate the continual release of particular enzymes and overload the body, thus a rotation diet should be followed with plenty of variety.[2,3,4]

The food should be balanced and contain a good mixture of carbohydrate, protein, essential fatty acids and fibre plus vitamins and minerals. Reducing the ingestion of sugar, yeast, dairy products and gluten usually helps, but, unless one is allergic to any of these, one should not completely eliminate them.

In the years that I have been treating CFS/ME, some of the weakest, most emaciated and immobile patients I have seen are those that have been following strict avoidance diets, often for many years. They usually start by being slightly intolerant of certain foods and within some months of avoiding those may become completely intolerant of many. As time goes on, more allergies seem to develop with the body's immune system going into 'free fall' mode and the patient rapidly descending into a form of allergic syndrome where almost every food, perfume, or deodorant causes adverse reactions.[5] My advice is that in the early stages if any food sensitivity has been discovered do not abstain totally for more than a month and, occasionally, eat a little of that substance.

Supplements

Vitamin and mineral supplements

These are widely recommended in the treatment of CFS/ME, but there is no evidence that mega doses of vitamins and minerals will relieve any of the CFS/ME symptoms. However, the antioxidant action of vitamin C has been shown to improve the body's immune response. With patients taking no more than 500 mg per day there have been no reported toxic side-effects. Similarly, the vitamin B group is known to improve the health of the nervous system. Functional deficiencies of the B vitamins pyridoxine, riboflavin and thiamine have been shown to occur in CFS/ME[7] and patients may therefore be advised to take one full and complete vitamin B-complex pill per day, provided that no complications are reported.

Some doctors specialising in CFS/ME give high doses of vitamin C and folic acid intravenously. I prescribe a 500 mg daily oral supplement of vitamin C and one complete vitamin B-complex pill to increase the patients' resistance to overall infection and improve the functioning of the nervous system.

Intramuscular injections of magnesium sulphate

This treatment is based on the belief that a magnesium deficiency is a primary cause of the disorder. Magnesium deficiency is associated with disorders of neuromuscular and psychiatric functioning. This deficiency results in an inability to cope with viral infections[8]. In 1991 a randomised controlled trial was conducted[9] that showed that 20 CFS/ME patients had significantly lower red blood cell magnesium levels compared with healthy controls. However, the benefits of taking extra magnesium for CFS/ME are still uncertain.[10]

Increased salt intake

Sodium deficiency can produce similar signs and symptoms to CFS/ME and is associated with low blood pressure. A form of low blood pressure that occurs as one stands up after sitting or lying (neurally mediated hypotension) frequently occurs in CFS/ME. However, the increase in salt intake that is occasionally advised may lead to severe, if not fatal, consequences for the many CFS/ME patients who suffer from high blood pressure.

Essential fatty acids

Central to the basis of the Perrin Technique is that in CFS/ME the hypothalmus is overactive leading to an overloaded autonomic system. Nerves transmit their signal via chemicals known as neurotransmitters. Too much of one of the main neurotransmitters, acetylcholine, breaks down into acetate and choline. Thus when originally formulating my theory in 1989 I hypothesised that one day scientists would discover too much choline in the body.

An increase of choline has indeed been found in the brain of CFS/ME sufferers by Professor Basant Puri of Hammersmith Hospital and Imperial College, London,[11] who has also discovered a deficiency in fatty acids which are important for the healthy maintenance of brain cell walls. This can be remedied by the intake of eicosapentaenoic acid (EPA), a constituent of certain fish oil supplements, which combines with the choline to heal the cell membranes and restore normal function of the brain. (This is fully explained in Professor Puri's book *Chronic Fatigue Syndrome – a natural way to treat M.E.* See further reading.)

Oral antifungals

The absence of the ultimate curative drug for CFS/ME has led to alternative approaches. In the late 1980s in Great Britain, one of the most popular hypotheses was that there is too much of the yeast Candida in the body as mentioned earlier in the chapter (pages 44–45). This causes many harmful effects,[12,] with recommended treatment usually by oral antifungals nystatin and ketoconazole, together with strict diets that prevent the forming of further Candida by excluding many foods.[1]

The use of antifungal agents in some patients has resulted in hepatitis[1,13] with many patients showing no improvements in CFS/ME symptoms. I have seen many patients who have had extensive tests that reveal no abnormal levels of Candida in their body, although they definitely suffer from CFS/ME.

Immunological therapies

The alternative term for CFS/ME in the USA is Chronic Fatigue and Immune Dysfunction Syndrome (CFIDS), an acknowledgement that dysfunction of the immune system is a major feature of the disease. Many immune modulatory treatments are expensive, not freely available, produce unpleasant side effects and yet yield inconclusive results (see Chapter 4).

Graded activity

Some psychologists believe that patients with CFS/ME 'perceive' greater fatigue during exercise as a result of the interaction of psychological distress, physical de-conditioning and/or sleep disturbance. They believe that the patient's fear of making their symptoms worse may lead to their reducing their activity and that the resultant physical de-conditioning can spiral into chronic disability, which leads to adverse psychological effects. Graded activity is the process of gently increasing in activity to counterbalance physical deconditioning. Patients are expected to follow the prescribed exercises, irrespective of any worsening in the symptoms and to fight against their 'perceived' fatigue.

The idea of graded exercise seems quite unsuitable to those patients who are struggling just to achieve basic activity at work or home. There is a ceiling, above which activity is counterproductive in many cases. Friedberg and Jason[14] advise exercise on an individual patient-by-patient basis, while many clinicians do not recommend it at all. However, significant improvement in functional capacity was noted in a year-long study in 1997[15] involving a graded exercise regime. Unfortunately, nearly half of the patients studied were taking antidepressants throughout the trial, which, in my view, undermines the validity of the study because as exercise has been shown to help in clinical depression it is likely that some of the patients who improved with exercise had been suffering from the latter rather than CFS/ME.

I believe that the reason why graded exercise has been shown to help in some cases is that, when the underlying disorder (CFS/ME) has receded, a patient who has been ill perhaps for many years may still be severely lacking in stamina. Exercise will improve the stamina, not the CFS/ME. It is important to understand the difference, as, if the graded activity is implemented too early in the patient's period of recovery, the illness will be exacerbated.

Exercise

Exercise often helps fatigue associated with an overall lack of fitness and with depression, but excessive activity always exacerbates fatigue in patients with CFS/ME. In fact, too much physical activity can trigger a relapse in someone who is on the road to recovery. The simple question every practitioner needs to ask when initially examining a possible CFS/ME patient is, 'Does exertion ever improve the symptoms or does it aggravate the condition'. If the latter is true, even if at the time of exertion the patient feels good, it is possibly CFS/ME.

If the patient feels occasionally improved following exercise, there could be an element of clinical depression. However, the patient may be suffering from both conditions at one time.

A positive approach is important in fighting any disorder, but the horrible irony of CFS/ME is that it usually affects people who are determined, positive characters who would usually beat most illnesses with will power alone. It is no secret that a strong will power has been shown to help combat all types of diseases, even some potentially fatal conditions such as cancer. The power of the mind appears to be a vital tool in overcoming pathology, probably by improving the immune system. However, the neurological pathway that is involved in this phenomenon is the sympathetic nervous system, the very system that breaks down in CFS/ME. Thus the more patients try to beat the illness by pushing themselves, the worse the symptoms may become. I usually recommend half the activity that the patient feels than s/he can cope with: if you feel able to walk 1 km, walk only 0.5 km. This is known as 'pacing'.

Together with the graded exercise programmes given out to most CFS/ME sufferers in UK hospital clinics comes advice about pacing.[16] As I have already noted, avoiding exercise due to a belief that it will exacerbate symptoms has been held responsible for maintaining symptoms in CFS/ME patients. However, significant improvement has been shown when patients are advised to avoid too much activity and carry out only 50 per cent of their perceived capabilities. In the early 1990s, when most of the medical fraternity were advocating exercise, exercise, exercise for CFS/ME, when patients who could hardly walk were advised to get fitter, I was telling all CFS/ME sufferers to stop and pace themselves, doing just half of whatever they felt they were capable of, whether it was walking, talking or watching TV. My Half Rule remains a major influence on the patient's overall improvement with my treatment. If the patient overdoes things during the course of treatment they may never fully recover; indeed, their health may worsen. Some patients tell me they find it difficult to gauge what half is. Often they have realised that they are doing too much after the particular activity and it is too late.

The best way of following the Half Rule is by thinking double. If you walk 0.5 km, ask yourself 'Can I honestly walk 1 km with no problem?' If the answer is no, 0.5 km is too much. If 1 km receives an emphatic yes with no worsening of the symptoms, 0.5 km is fine. If you are uncertain, even 0.5 km may be too much and you should reduce the distance. The same applies to any activity, for example, having a conversation: if half an hour is too much, engage in only ten-minute chats at one time. If a two-hour film is too long, use a video recorder in order to watch half-hour sections at a time, provided that you feel you could watch an hour without adverse effects. This prevents you from overstressing your sympathetic nervous system and, although it is difficult to implement, I have found this to be the golden rule that may be the difference between helping some patients and completely curing them.

Cognitive behavioural therapy

The effectiveness of cognitive behavioural therapy (CBT) in the treatment of CFS/ME has been comprehensively reviewed.[17–20] It has been shown to be more effective when delivered by properly trained clinicians in specialised clinics.[17] CBT is based on the belief that psychological factors are maintaining CFS/ME in all patients. Such factors may include faulty beliefs, ineffective coping behaviour and negative mood states.[19] Distorted thought patterns may lead to anxiety and depression.[18]

My view is that the depression and anxiety often seen in CFS/ME sufferers are secondary to the underlying physical symptoms of CFS/ME. Depression and anxiety create a heightened sense of frustration and guilt in the patient who in any case feels himself to be a heavy burden on family and friends. Those people, including health care providers, who do not acknowledge the existence of CFS/ME, may exacerbate this frustration. However, CBT may help the patient to deal with secondary feelings of guilt and worthlessness.

In a 1996 randomised study[20] on CFS/ME patients diagnosed using the Oxford criteria (see Chapter 2), the group receiving CBT were functionally improved, but many reported continuing fatigue. However, in a separate study reported four years later, patients in the CBT group demonstrated significant improvements in physical functioning and substantial reductions in fatigue.[21] Some patients in the latter[21] study had a current psychiatric diagnosis and others were receiving additional antidepressant therapy. It is probable that CFS/ME patients who have difficulty in coping with their illness will benefit from CBT. In common with other chronic illnesses, positive coping strategies and lifestyle management approaches may reduce the depression and anxiety levels, but there is little evidence that CBT has a significant effect on other symptoms of the illness. It is worth noting that while many of the patients helped by CBT in the 1996[20] study were also suffering from a diagnosed psychiatric illness, in another study on CBT where the CFS/ME patients were diagnosed using a different Australian system of criteria, which excluded psychiatric diagnosis, few differences were noted between the CBT treatment group and the controls who did not receive the CBT.[22]

Antidepressants

Treatment of the musculoskeletal disorder, fibrositis, involves the use of antidepressants together with anti-inflammatory drugs.[23] This treatment has been clinically shown to help the muscular pain in that condition. The soreness in fibrositis resembles the pain in some CFS/ME cases and, accordingly, similar treatment has been advocated.[23,24]

Low doses of antidepressants have been shown to improve the sleep patterns of some patients.[25] However, some older antidepressants are habit-forming and may result in significant physical and psychological side effects, while certain foods have to be avoided while taking these older antidepressants as they can cause harmful reactions. There are fewer such problems with today's antidepressants. However, if you are prescribed medication that aggravates your symptoms, you should return to your doctor to discuss the option of an alternative antidepressant. This is the same for all pharmaceutical approaches to treatment, including herbal remedies. In other words, if a drug reduces one or more of the symptoms with no major side effect, it may prove helpful in the battle against CFS/ME. However, if the reaction to the medicine outweighs the overall benefit or if it worsens the symptoms, you should immediately consult your GP or specialist in order to review the alternatives.

Hypnosis

Hypnosis has been tested in a pilot study[26] on CFS/ME patients who reported that hypnosis helped in muscle pain management both at rest and after exertion with a slight improvement in quality of life, but there was no increase in cognitive ability.

A lasting cure

Two complex problems beset the diagnosis and treatment of CFS/ME. The first is that two conditions – or more – can exist at any one time in one patient. It is sometimes difficult, for example, to distinguish between depression and CFS/ME, particularly in those cases of CFS/ME in which depression is an additional feature. The second problem is that because there is no accepted means of diagnosis, by tests such as blood or urine analysis, most doctors diagnose CFS/ME **by exclusion**. In other words, the patient will be diagnosed as suffering from CFS/ME only when all other possible diagnoses have been excluded (see Chapter 6). In my view, this is a hazardous method of diagnosing any disease. Can you imagine if a doctor were to tell a patient, "Well, after all the tests, we cannot find anything else wrong with you, so it must be cancer". Yet thousands of people around the world are being told that they have CFS/ME, using the exclusion method of diagnosis.

Some medical experts on CFS/ME have touched upon the neurological effects of the disease, and how the immune system and the body's hormones are affected.

However, the treatment recommended by these specialists is to improve the hormonal and chemical balance by dietary means and, if necessary, by psychiatric drugs or psychotherapy. These treatments do help in many cases, but I believe that these experts are missing a crucial point: in my view, they are treating the symptoms rather than the root cause of the disease.

The neurological system that controls the hormonal and chemical balance of the body is the autonomic nervous system and the system that is the main factor in drainage of poisons from the body is the lymphatic system. If these two systems were working correctly, the body would cope with extra stresses and strains after being detoxified or desensitised. Only then might psychotherapy help, and a healthy hypoallergenic diet might bring about a permanent improvement in patients with CFS/ME.

Sadly, in many people with CFS/ME there is little or no recovery, despite many and varied dietary and chemical approaches to treatment.

The key is to find a complete and lasting cure that helps the body cope with extra stress, rather than temporarily reducing the symptoms. This concept is in keeping with modern medicine's approach to the management of other types of disease. For example, the use of vaccinations to increase the body's antibodies, and thus resist certain types of infections.

If one regards any stress factor as the infection, the obvious course of action is to increase the body's defence in staving off the infection. The fortification of the body is controlled by the autonomic nervous system, particularly the sympathetic nerves. This elaborate web of nerve tissue stems from the middle section of the spine, and spreads throughout the body (see Chapter 3). As already stated in Chapter 3, American neurophysiologist, Dr Irvin M. Korr, made a lifetime study of the autonomic nerves,[27–33] and how mechanical stimulation of this system has a major effect on the body as a whole. My treatment programme and my theory as to the cause of CFS/ME, which is described in detail in later chapters, is influenced greatly by the work of this scientist who was a luminary of osteopathic philosophy.

Many sportsmen and women – such as Mr E, described at the start of Chapter 1 – exert more strain upon their dorsal (upper) spine in the pursuit of their sport than the average individual. Golf, yachting, cycling, tennis and weight-lifting are just a few different types of sports that put extra stress on the upper back. In some individuals this could lead to irritation of the sympathetic nervous system, resulting in the development of CFS/ME.

Since the early 1990s people suffering from this debilitating disorder have arrived at my practices in the North-west and South-east of England, desperate for help and a sympathetic ear. At first I thought it unlikely that I would be able to help, but, as more patients came, I began to notice a familiar pattern. There were common postural and mechanical factors shared by the patients. These similarities, consequently, led to the establishment of my manual system of diagnosis and treatment for this disease.

The case of Mr J

Age: 19 years
Occupation: Law student
Marital status: Single

Originally I knew Mr J socially. We saw each other at a party where he told me that he had been forced to take time off from college due to ill health.

He explained that he had initially suffered from a viral infection six months earlier. Since then, he had felt very lethargic, complaining of aches in all his limbs and palpitations. His symptoms were aggravated by exertion. His doctor had diagnosed ME and he enquired whether I had heard of it.

I told him of my research and the fact that I was writing a book about the subject. A few days later, the young man was lying on my treatment table, hoping for me to perform miracles. He had been convinced nobody could help him and that he just had to rest at home until he felt well enough to return to his studies. I knew that my methods had worked on others, and was genuinely convinced that I could treat him successfully.

His dorsal spine was restricted and his posture was typical of a student who bent over his books at home, and slouched in a lecture hall during the day.

After nine treatment sessions over four months Mr J returned to college, almost back to normal, and his symptoms of CFS/ME had abated. Through a chance meeting at a party he was able to return to healthy, active life. Now he is a successful city lawyer with a large family and he has been symptom-free for over ten years.

Chapter 6

Defining fatigue

> Life is one long process of getting tired.
>
> *Samuel Butler (1835–1902)*

What do we mean by the term 'fatigue'? According to the *Oxford English Dictionary* definition, fatigue is 'Lassitude or weariness resulting from either bodily or mental exertion. Physiologically as: A condition of muscles, organs or cells characterised by a temporary reduction in power or sensitivity following a period of prolonged activity or stimulation.'

Patients tend to express their feelings of fatigue as aches in muscles, severe pain in joints, weakness in one or more limb, and/or a lack of energy and vitality. Patients with CFS/ME may feel as though they have just run a marathon when they have only walked round the block, or that picking up their suitcase is as hard a task as trying to lift a ton weight. In other words, the resultant aches and pains are apparently unjustified in relation to the physical stress on the body.

What happens in fatigue

Muscle fibres contract due to stimulation from the nerves known as motor nerves. These motor nerves form part of the somatic nervous system, which is involved in the control of voluntary movements within the body. When over-exercising individual muscles, the contractile power within the muscle fibres is eventually depleted until a state of fatigue develops. This loss of power may be caused by a breakdown at different stages of the muscle-reflex pathway. In other words, there could be a failure in the transmission of somatic nerve impulses to the muscle, or there could be a collapse in the actual contractile mechanism inside the muscle.

Causes other than CFS/ME

Fatigue is often regarded by practitioners as being psychogenic (all in the mind) in origin. It may, of course, result from severe physical and/or mental activity, or lack of sleep. The degree of the fatigue will vary according to the personality and stamina of the individual.

Experiments have shown that if a movement of the hand is continued for long enough to initiate a state of fatigue, and if at this stage the blood flow into the hand is stopped by inflating a cuff around the upper arm, although the somatic motor nerves are still functioning, there is no recovery of power until the cuff is released and normal circulation is restored.[1] As mentioned in chapter 3, the blood flow to muscles is under the influence of the sympathetic nervous system. Thus, if the sympathetic nerves are not functioning correctly, blood flow to certain muscles could be reduced. One could then reasonably assume that these muscles would be likely to suffer from some form of fatigue.

My work indicates that in CFS/ME normal activity within the sympathetic nervous system breaks down. The effect may be systemic, causing widespread aches and pains in the entire body, or the fatigue may be limited to one or two muscle groups.

As other disorders can cause fatigue symptoms. CFS/ME is generally judged to be the cause of fatigue only when these other diseases have been ruled out, and all other possible explanations have been explored. Although CFS/ME is a possibility in all cases of fatigue, it is good practice always to ensure that no other serious condition is at the root of the problem.

Anaemia

Lack of oxygen to the tissues of the body leads to fatigue. This happens if there is a reduction in the oxygen-carrying red blood cells, or the function of these cells becomes impaired, as in some cases of anaemia, a major symptom being that of lethargy and weakness. A common cause of anaemia is iron deficiency, since iron is the main constituent of the oxygen-transporting element (haemoglobin) within red blood cells. A simple blood test to determine the level of iron, or a red blood cell count will eliminate anaemia from the doctor's investigation.

Heart conditions

Heart problems may lead to impaired blood flow to the rest of the body, which, subsequently, will lead to a reduced supply of nutrients and oxygen. This in turn will cause feelings of fatigue. Since pains in the chest and arms, as well as increased heart rate, are common signs and symptoms of heart disorders, the sufferer will often interpret these signs as an impending heart attack. However, these symptoms are very common in CFS/ME. After listening to the patient's heart and running other tests, such as an electrocardiogram (ECG), the doctor should be in a position to discount heart disease as the cause of the problem. I have seen some CFS/ME patients in a serious state of anxiety over their chest pains and palpitations as in the case of Mr C (see Chapter 3). Practitioners should be aware of the distress these symptoms cause and ensure the patient is satisfied that a cardiac arrest is not imminent.

Lung disorders

Oxygen depletion occurs if the lungs are not functioning correctly. This will result in fatigue within the muscles and since CFS/ME can leave a person feeling breathless, lung function, as well as heart rhythms, should be thoroughly investigated.

Bowel and kidney disorders

These should be eliminated from the investigation, as the resultant metabolic changes that can occur may lead to fatigue.

Glandular fever

One specific disease that is frequently mistaken for CFS/ME, and vice versa, is infectious mononucleosis (better known as glandular fever), due to infection by the Epstein-Barr virus. An analysis of the blood will reveal a large increase in mononuclear, agranular white cells. A specific blood test, known as the Paul Bunnell test, will confirm if the signs and symptoms are caused by glandular fever. The test is readily available at your family doctor's.

Addison's disease

This disorder, which can cause fatigue, plagued American president John F. Kennedy (1917–1963), for much of his life. Addison's disease is due to a disturbance in the normal function of the adrenal glands, situated next to the kidneys. The dysfunction leads to a deficiency of the hormones produced by the adrenals. The condition is improved by hormone replacement therapy and, often, steroids.

Patients with Addison's disease usually present with muscle wasting and a darkened pigmentation of the skin. Their blood pressure is often lowered and sufferers may lose their appetite and experience nausea and vomiting. Although there are some similarities between this disease and CFS/ME, the skin discoloration, a drop in the serum levels of the adreno-cortical hormones and a fall in blood pressure are all signs of Addison's that are easily detectable by clinical tests.

Myasthenia gravis

Nerves transmit their impulses by means of chemicals known as neurotransmitter substances. When a motor nerve, which controls muscles, enters the muscle fibre, it releases the transmitter substance, acetylcholine, which stimulates the fibre to contract. In the rare disease myasthenia gravis, which affects mostly young women, there is a disturbance in the production of acetylcholine, which results in a marked weakness in the muscles. The patient feels this frailty especially at the end of the day. The muscles in the head are often affected first, causing difficulty in swallowing and chewing. The eyelids become very heavy and even holding up the head can become arduous. The muscular weakness in myasthenia gravis can be quickly relieved by the administration of certain medications, such as endrophonium chloride. The rapid improvement is the key to establishing the diagnosis. As discussed in Chapter 5, during the early stages of CFS/ME there is often an overproduction of acetylcholine in the brain leading to too much choline.[2]

Gilbert's syndrome

This benign hereditary disorder, another cause of fatigue, is associated with an excess amount of bile pigment in the blood, known as bilirubin. Gilbert's syndrome is characterised by mild, intermittent jaundice, occasional bowel disturbances and often by weakness and fatigue. A simple blood test will confirm whether or not the patient's fatigue is caused by this disorder.

Infection

Chronic infections, such as toxoplasmosis, an infection caused by a microscopic parasite that can live inside the cells of humans and animals, especially cats and farm animals, should be eliminated in the diagnostic process. Diagnosis of toxoplasmosis is usually conducted through blood tests.

Lyme disease is an infection that originates from a tick bite. The disease has a variety of symptoms, including changes affecting the skin, heart, joints and nervous system. It is also known as borrelia or borreliosis. A diagnosis of Lyme disease is more likely if the patient can remember a tick bite and has the characteristic erythema migrans rash.

To make a diagnosis the doctor may take a blood sample to determine whether or not the patient has developed an antibody towards Lyme disease. However, a live blood analysis, preferred by some physicians, is more accurate.

Early stages of HIV infection may resemble symptoms of CFS/ME and should be ruled out by a blood test.

Hormonal disorders

In CFS/ME it is very common for hormonal levels to be slightly higher or lower than normal and this is due, primarily, to the hypothalamus not functioning correctly. Many other primary hormonal disorders, such as hypothyroidism, thyrotoxicosis, diabetes mellitus and hyperparathyroidism, may cause symptoms common to CFS/ME. These disorders can be verified by means of blood tests.

Thyroid function tests should be carried out to monitor the production of thyroxine (T4) and triiodothyronine (T3) in the thyroid gland. Thyroid-releasing hormone (TRH) is secreted by the hypothalamus and stimulates the production of thyroid-stimulating hormone (TSH) from the anterior pituitary gland. TSH in turn stimulates the production and release of T4 and T3 from the thyroid. Blood tests for TSH, T3 and T4 should be done in order to verify that the thyroid is functioning correctly.

Neuromuscular disorders

Neuromuscular diseases such as multiple sclerosis (MS), a disorder that affects the central nervous system, should be eliminated as a possible cause of fatigue. MS, also known as disseminated sclerosis, is a chronic, inflammatory disease that can cause a variety of symptoms, including changes in sensation, visual problems, muscle weakness, depression, difficulties with coordination and speech, severe fatigue and pain. A fatty layer, known as the myelin sheath, surrounds and protects some nerves: this layer helps the nerves carry electrical signals. In MS the myelin is gradually destroyed, in patches, throughout the brain and spinal cord, causing a variety of symptoms, depending upon which signals are interrupted. MS can usually be detected by MRI scans and analysis of cerebrospinal fluid taken by means of a lumbar puncture. A number of other neuromuscular disorders can also cause fatigue.

Tumours

Malignant disease such as undiagnosed lymphomas and other tumours should be ruled out by investigations such as blood tests and, when necessary, scans such as MRI.

Auto-immune diseases

Diseases of the immune system, such as rheumatoid arthritis and systemic lupus erythematosus (SLE), are important to consider when diagnosing CFS/ME. SLE is a chronic, autoimmune disease of the joints, skin, kidney, brain, heart, lungs and gastrointestinal tract. It occurs mostly in women of childbearing age. While SLE patients usually have joint swelling and pain, CFS/ME patients may suffer painful joints but they do not usually experience swelling. A characteristic redness on the cheeks and nose of patients, the so-called 'butterfly rash', hair loss and a history of multiple miscarriages are all symptoms of SLE; however, some CFS/ME cases have similar symptoms. Blood tests can identify the antibodies produced in autoimmune diseases.

More than one disease

This chapter demonstrates just a few of the many other origins of fatigue and shows that only by comprehensive tests can other possibilities be eliminated from the investigation. However, even if tests show other reasons for the symptoms, it does not necessarily exclude the diagnosis of CFS/ME. It continues to worry me how many CFS/ME patients are diagnosed primarily by the exclusion of other better understood diseases. It is perfectly possible, and common, for people to suffer more than one disease or disorder at one time.

In my years of research and treating hundreds of sufferers since the early 1990s, I have observed physical signs, time and again, that are common to all CFS/ME patients. These signs, which are discussed in detail later in the book, can be detected by any trained practitioner and provide a much needed aid in diagnosis.

The case of Miss L

Age: 12 years
Occupation: school student

This case illustrates the diagnostic confusion that surrounds CFS/ME. Miss L had been severely disabled with an unknown disorder for the previous eighteen months. She had been wheelchair-bound for some of the time and unable to attend her regular school for more than a few hours a week. She had mostly spent the day at home, cared for by her devoted single mother, who had two other young daughters to look after. She had been taken to a local health authority school for a few hours each week; even that had often been too taxing for her ailing body.

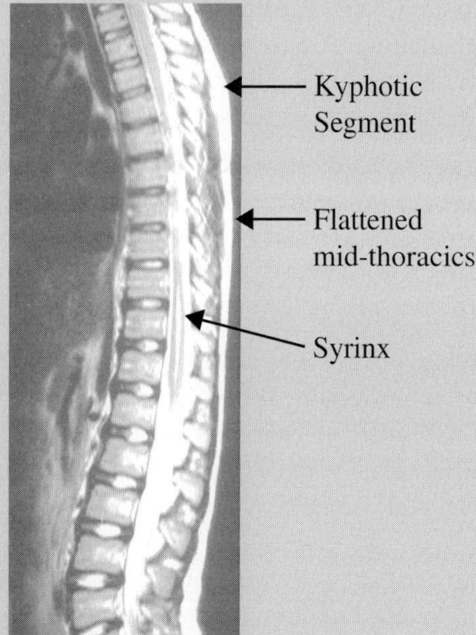

Figure 7. *MRI sagittal image showing spinal defect in 12 year old girl with CFS/ME.*
The postural disturbance of the thoracic spine in most cases of CFS/ME is usually not too severe with usual evidence of old osteochondrosis with a flattened upper thoracic region. A syrinx (cyst within the spinal canal) seen in this MR image is rare but demonstrates the extent of possible spinal dysfunction.

Miss L was born with a syrinx in the middle of her spine (see Fig. 7). A syrinx is a cyst that forms within the spinal cord and usually leads to a condition known as syringiomyelia. This neurological condition leads to a loss of pain sensation and reduction of normal sensory function on one side of the body, in other words, a different set of symptoms to CFS/ME. Miss L also had a defect at the top of her neck. A small section of her brain was slightly protruding down into the spinal canal (see Fig. 8). When this latter condition is severe, it is known as a Chiari malformation and is responsible for many symptoms common to CFS/ME as it affects normal spinal cord function. Chiari malformation often presents in a patient who also has a syrinx.

Cases of Chiari malformation and cervical stenosis, in which the spinal canal has narrowed and the health and function of the spinal cord are compromised, have been observed in CFS/ME patients.[3]

Miss L had two conditions that could have caused major neurological problems, but her symptoms, which included severe fatigue, headache, lack of concentration, sleep disturbance, irritable bowel and irritable bladder, sore throat and pains in her neck, back, chest and extremities, were diagnosed at

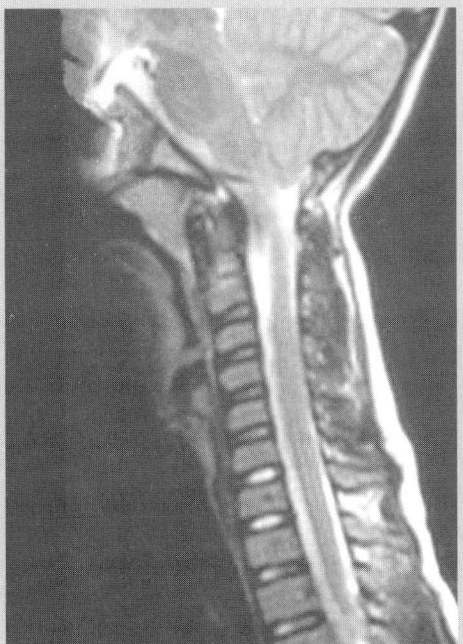

Figure 8. *Upper cervical defect in the same 12 year old girl.*
A defect at the uppermost region of the cervical spine is found in many cases of CFS/ME. The sagittal MR scan shows a partial herniation of the cerebellar tonsil into the spinal canal. (If the herniation penetrates further into the cervical region it is known as a Chiari Malformation).

her local hospital as mostly psychological. The syrinx, in their opinion, had nothing to do with the symptoms and the upper spine problem was not severe enough to be classified as a Chiari malformation and was considered to be unrelated to her condition. CFS/ME was never mentioned and when her mother brought her in to see me, I found it difficult to believe that the only treatment Miss L was receiving was regular sessions with the hospital psychologist. Miss L's paediatric neurologist dismissed the idea that she had CFS/ME. However, as her treatment slowly progressed and her symptoms started to improve, Miss L's doctors began to take notice. I explained to them how the girl's spine was extremely flattened in the upper part of her back. Her breastbone was slightly malformed, showing a slight concavity, which would have affected her respiratory mechanics. She had lymphatic swelling in her chest and neck as well as the tender areas familiar to all the CFS/ME patients that I had seen (see Chapter 8). Although Miss L's doctors continued to be sceptical, they could see the encouraging results my treatment and they then included me in Miss L's case-management meetings at the hospital.

Miss L eventually restarted mainstream school and at the time of writing no longer needs the wheelchair. She is at present a very active 15 year old with a full life. Even though she had other health issues, the main cause of her symptoms was restricted lymphatic drainage aggravated by her syrinx and upper neck malformation. This was evident in the response to my treatment. The hospital neurologist has discharged her and she now comes to me for check-ups every couple of months.

Chapter 7

The significance of toxins in CFS/ME

What is food to one, is to others bitter poison.

Lucretius (96 BC–55 BC)

The word toxin was coined in the late nineteenth century and is defined as an antigenic poison or venom of plant or animal origin, especially one produced or derived from micro-organisms and causing disease when present at low concentrations in the body (*The New Oxford Dictionary of English*, 2001). For simplicity 'toxin' is used in this book in the broader sense of any substance that is harmful to the body. Accordingly, mercury, which is a heavy metal toxin, is from neither plant nor animal source but it is nevertheless a major toxin to the body.

Pollutants

Environmental pollutants have long been seen as major causative factors in neurodegenerative disorders such as Parkinson's disease, although there may also be genetic factors that make a person more susceptible to that illness.[1] Studies[2] have revealed major variations in an individual's ability to detoxify noxious agents and have shown that neurological disease may derive from an exceptional vulnerability to certain neurotoxins. This susceptibility is from both external sources in the environment and from free radicals (see Chapter 4) and toxic chemicals normally found within the central nervous system.

A few examples of the different types of toxins are listed in this chapter. However, over 60,000 chemicals were identified in the 1990s as known or potential toxic substances by the United States Environmental Protection Agency.[3] The US Government Office of Technology estimated that up to 25 per cent of all chemicals might be neurotoxic.[4] Each year approximately 1000 new chemicals are produced and, no matter what safety procedures are taken, they are all – inadvertently or deliberately – introduced into the environment via the air, water or foodstuffs.[5] There are eight basic sources of toxic exposure, most of which have been implicated as potential causative factors of CFS/ME:[6,7,8 9,10]

1. Air pollutants (indoor and outdoor):
   - benzene
   - chloroform
   - CFCs, PCBs
   - tobacco smoke
2. Food contaminants and additives:
   - cadmium
   - aspartame (E951)
3. Water pollutants:
   - heavy metals, such as lead, mercury and aluminium
4. Soil contaminants:
   - pesticides such as chlordane, DDT and other organophosphates
5. Chemicals used in hobbies and crafts:
   - trichloroethane
6. Chemicals used in household activities:
   - methylene chloride
7. Workplace contaminants:
   - toluene
   - solvents
   - radiation
8. Environmental accidents and wars.
9. Vaccinations and Gulf War Syndrome.

1. Air pollutants (indoor and outdoor)

Benzene is a widely used chemical and is one of the top 20 chemicals by production volume in the USA. Outdoor air contains low levels of benzene from tobacco smoke, automobile service stations, exhaust from motor vehicles and industrial emissions. People may breathe in vapours from products that contain benzene, such as glues, paints, furniture wax and detergents. Breathing benzene can cause drowsiness, dizziness and unconsciousness; long-term benzene exposure affects the bone marrow and can cause anaemia and leukaemia.[11]

Chloroform is a colourless liquid with a pleasant, non-irritating odour and a slightly sweet taste. In the past, chloroform was used as an inhaled anaesthetic pre-surgery, but it is not used in that way today. Chloroform is used to make other chemicals and is formed in small amounts when chlorine is added to water. Other names for chloroform include trichloromethane and methyl trichloride. People are exposed to chloroform when breathing contaminated air and when drinking or touching the substance or water that contains it. Breathing chloroform can cause dizziness, fatigue and headaches and long-term exposure may damage the liver and kidneys. It can cause sores if large amounts touch the skin.[12]

Chlorofluorocarbons (CFCs) are chemical compounds, consisting of gases, such as methane or ethane combined with both chlorine and fluorine. They were formerly widely used in industry, for example as refrigerants, propellants and cleaning solvents. Their use has been prohibited as they have been held responsible for part of the depletion of the ozone layer and are now substituted by hydrochlorofluorocarbons (HCFCs) – which are now believed to cause liver disease.[13.]

Polychlorinated biphenyls (PCBs) are a class of organic compounds with 1 to 10 chlorine atoms attached to biphenyl, which contains benzene (see above). PCB mixtures have been used for a variety of applications, including hydraulic fluids, lubricating and cutting oil, and as additives in pesticides, paints, adhesives and plastics. People exposed to large amounts of PCBs suffer skin conditions such as rashes. Studies in exposed workers have shown possible liver damage.[14]

Tobacco smoke contains nicotine, which is a stimulant of the nervous system leading to addiction. Medical research has determined that tobacco smoke together with its tar is a major contributing factor towards many health problems, particularly lung cancer, emphysema, and cardiovascular disease.[17]

2. Food contaminants and additives

Cadmium is a naturally occurring metallic element and present everywhere in our environment. Cadmium was first used in industrial batteries and as coatings for the protection of steel from corrosion. Under normal conditions, adverse human health effects have not been seen in the general population. However, long-term occupational exposure can cause severe adverse health effects on the internal organs.[18]

Aspartame is an artificial, non-carbohydrate sweetener (aspartyl-phenylalanine-1-methyl ester). It is commonly used in diet soft drinks and is often provided as a table condiment. In the European Union, it is also known under the E number (additive code) E951. Aspartame is one of the sugar substitutes used by diabetics. Yet, along with other food additives and colourants such as Brilliant Blue and Quinoline Yellow, aspartame has been shown to have neurotoxic properties.[19]

3. Water pollutants

Heavy metals

The doses of neurotoxins required to produce behavioural and/or sensory dysfunctions are low and may be cumulative, as for example with methylmercury exposure in adults.[21] The nervous system may be particularly vulnerable during fetal development. Toxicants such as ethanol may exert their greatest effect *in utero* while others, such as **lead**, produce IQ defects in children.[22] It has been suggested that heavy metal toxins pass to the infant via the mother's breast milk and that higher concentrations of toxicity transfer to the older child, particularly the firstborn if breast-fed.[23]

Mercury has been implicated as a major heavy metal neurotoxin, leading to neurological dysfunction and oxidative stress. A primary source of mercury poisoning is the amalgam in dental fillings.[24] CFS/ME sufferers should be tested for mercury content in the blood. If it is high, seek out a dentist expert in replacing amalgam fillings. The most likely time during which mercury can enter the blood is during the process of inserting or extracting the filling. The procedure must therefore be carried out with the necessary safety precautions in place. It is equally important that when any local anaesthetic is injected in the mouth it should be non-adrenaline based. The usual anaesthetics administered by dentists contain adrenaline, which will over-stimulate the sympathetic nervous system and could have a disastrous effect on CFS/ME sufferers.

Long before the issues concerning MMR were raised, mercury poisoning had been implicated in problems with vaccinations. Mercury is present in the preservative thiomersal, a component of vaccinations. Vaccinations against cholera, tetanus, typhoid and influenza have been implicated as causative factors of CFS/ME.[25]

Other heavy metals such as **aluminium** have been shown, like mercury, to exert neurotoxic effects and thus could be a major factor in the disease process in some CFS/ME patients.[26]

4. Soil contaminants

As early as 1961 chronic fatigue was seen as a major symptom following long term exposure to **organophosphates**,[27] so it is no surprise that levels of serum organochlorides have been found to be higher in CFS/ME patients compared with normal subjects.[28]

Chlordane is a man-made pesticide, used from 1948, that leads to toxic exposure of farm workers, gardeners and pest control workers. Even though it has been banned in the USA since 1988, chlordane is still found, many years later, in the air of homes treated for termites. Most health effects in humans that may be linked to chlordane exposure are on the nervous system, the digestive system, the liver and the immune system.[20]

5. Chemicals used in hobbies and crafts

Trichloroethane has been used over the years as a general solvent, particularly for degreasing. Exposure to trichloroethane usually occurs by breathing contaminated air. It is found in building materials, cleaning products, paints and metal degreasing agents. Long-term exposure can lead to disease of the liver.[29]

6. Chemicals used in household activities

Aerosol propellants found in hair spray, deodorants and spray paints contain high levels of **methylene chloride**, which, when inhaled, affects the brain and liver, causing symptoms such as fatigue, lethargy, headaches and chest pain. Analysis of the breath in residents in a New Jersey suburb in the States revealed traces of many toxic compounds, including chloroform, benzene, carbon tetrachloride, trichlorethane and other harmful pollutants.[30]

7. Workplace contaminants

Toluene, also known as methylbenzene or phenylmethane, is used as an industrial feedstock and as a solvent. It is a clear, colourless liquid, which is found mainly in crude oil. It is also produced when making coke from coal. It causes disturbance of the nervous system. People are often affected by breathing in contaminated workplace air, automobile exhaust fumes, some paints, paint thinners, nail varnish, lacquers and adhesives.[15,16]

Most causes of toxicity that can affect the work place such as the solvent trichloroethane have already been discussed in this chapter.[29] However, in the present era, we are exposed to invisible agents as well as the discernible. **Radiation** exposure can cause the release of a range of toxic compounds in damaged tissue. A survey of 11,000 Norwegians and Swedes found that many were suffering headaches and fatigue from using mobile phones. Risk of brain tumours in the temporal lobe has been shown to be increased by the use of the analogue cellular mobile phones on the same side as the tumour.[31] Scientists working for the Radiation and Nuclear Safety Authority in Finland have found that exposing humans to one hour of mobile phone radiation affected the integrity of the blood-brain barrier, leading to larger toxic molecules passing into the CSF, with the potential of causing damage to brain tissue.[32]

8. Environmental accidents and wars

Major environmental disasters occasionally occur – such as the sinking of an oil tanker, or a pipeline rupture that kills many fish and birds and, sometimes, harms entire ecosystems. However, in recent times one of the worst ecological black spots has been Kuwait during the First Gulf War (1990–1991), where millions of gallons of crude oil were pumped into the sea and part of an entire oil field was set alight. This has been associated with Gulf War Syndrome which shares many symptoms with CFS/ME.

9. Vaccinations and Gulf War Syndrome

Vaccines are clearly associated with Gulf War Syndrome, which shares many symptoms with CFS/ME.[33,34] Central as well as peripheral nervous system dysfunction occurred in the veterans of the first Gulf War (GWVs) who were exposed to both chemical and severe psychological war stresses.[35,36] However, environmental factors could also be responsible for some of the disorders seen in GWVs.[37]

Exposure to pesticides (particularly organophosphates), oil and smoke from the oil well fires, depleted uranium, as well as vaccines, could all have contributed to the many cases of acute and chronic respiratory illnesses reported in GWVs. In fact as many as 70 per cent of those receiving two or more vaccines, given simultaneously during deployment, showed signs of acute or chronic respiratory illnesses. The war to free Kuwait from the invading forces of Iraq (1990–1991) has been described as the most toxic war in western military history,[38] with at least 14 per cent of US GWVs fulfilling the CDC criteria of chronic fatigue syndrome[39] (see Chapter 2).

The research on GWVs has yielded another important conclusion: post-traumatic stress disorder was not a major factor and that any soldiers diagnosed with this psychological disorder were mostly ill before deployment – at the time when vaccinations were at their highest level. In fact, occurrences of post-traumatic stress disorder lessened during deployment.[40,41] This throws doubt on suggestions that GWVs are simply suffering from a psychiatric war syndrome.

Effects of neurotoxins

Toxic chemical exposure can cause many serious conditions, including cardiovascular, kidney and endocrine diseases, depression and psychosis. The most common organ to be affected by toxins is the brain, leading to fatigue, exhaustion, cognitive impairment, loss of memory, insomnia and other disturbing symptoms.[42]

There are several specialised regions of the brain's ventricular system, termed circumventricular organs, which interact closely with the cerebrospinal fluid. These zones are chemical-sensitive regions that may react with toxins, sending messages to other parts of the brain, especially the hypothalamus.

The hypothalamus controls the hormonal system via a mechanism called biofeedback. Basically, the hypothalamus 'tastes' the blood to check how much hormone needs to be released into the circulation. It then sends messages to endocrine organs around the body to increase or decrease the many different hormonal levels. Since hormones are made up of large protein molecules, the blood-brain barrier, which normally protects against large toxic molecules, does not function in the region of the hypothalamus. Thus the most permeable region of the blood brain barrier is at the hypothalamus, facilitating its ability to monitor hormone levels in the blood. This increased permeability, together with the aforementioned messages from these receptor sites, makes the hypothalamus the most vulnerable region in the brain to suffer a toxic insult from large molecular chemicals, such as cytokines and opioid peptides mentioned in Chapter 4.

Autonomic dysfunction has long been associated with many toxic substances especially following exposure to organic solvents, with some people exhibiting signs and symptoms of peripheral neuropathy.

Under normal conditions, the blood-brain barrier protects the central nervous system from rapid fluctuations in levels of ions, neurotransmitters, bacterial toxins, growth factors and other substances. The permeability of the blood-brain barrier has been shown to be increased by stress.[43]

Each organ or tissue may act as a discreet target for some toxic substances, which may lead to dysfunction of the whole organism. Specific molecules within a particular cell type act as primary targets. Some neurons are less susceptible to toxic damage, leading to regions of the brain that are not as sensitive to toxins.

Excess amounts of the neurotransmitter, acetylcholine, could eventually lead to high levels of choline in the brain. Some toxins irreversibly inhibit the action of enzymes that break down this chemical transmitter, leading to a surplus of acetylcholine, which becomes toxic to the nervous system. This has been seen[44] in the organophosphate-exposed patients who served in the first Gulf War (1990–1991). As discussed in Chapter 5, an increase in choline has been discovered in CFS/ME.[45]

Diet and toxicity

Exposure to chemicals affects people in different ways depending on several factors. Diet plays a crucial part in the body's ability to withstand toxicity. Toxins can be produced from non-toxic foods that we eat, building up in the central nervous system, liver or kidneys. Sugar may not be broken down correctly when energy is required, leading to brain and muscle fatigue and many other signs and symptoms.

Trace elements, which are often used as supplements for good health, may become toxic if ingested in too high a dose. One thinks of selenium, for example, as a promoter of health, but it may be taken up from the soil by certain plants such as species of the *Astralagus* genus in sufficient quantities to render those plants toxic. Chronic selenium poisoning in animals, known as alkali disease, leads to cases of livestock with lameness, lack of vitality, hair loss, depressed appetite and emaciation.[46]

Healthy food may not be properly digested or absorbed. A leaky gut due to injury of the intestinal wall may be present, leading to semi-digested food entering the bloodstream,[47,48] causing immune responses, which create further toxicity.

Damage to the lining of the alimentary canal may be caused by a variety of irritants, most common being alcohol, aspirin, gluten and *Candida albicans*.[49] Deficiencies in some vitamins, proteins, essential fatty acids and minerals are known to lead to poor intestinal cell growth, causing increased permeability of the gut wall.[50]

Predisposition to toxicity

Previous exposure to toxins will increase an individual's sensitivity to further toxic insult. Some people have a greater genetic ability to detoxify while, unfortunately, others are more likely to experience more severe symptoms from toxic causes due to their individual genetic predisposition. Likewise, prior state of health, with the emphasis on the immune system, is a major significant factor to consider when assessing human ability to withstand exposure to poisonous chemicals. Age is important, with children much more susceptible to toxic overload than adults, because of their faster rate of absorption and smaller body weight – hence the smaller dosages of prescribed medicine allowed to children.[51]

Several chemicals have the potential to induce autoimmune diseases [52,53,54] such as systemic lupus erythematosus, commonly known as lupus or SLE. Genetic susceptibilities have been discovered in diseases such as autoimmune hepatitis.[55] I believe that the immune profile seen in some CFS/ME sufferers is likely to render these individuals more prone to toxic attack; however, much more research is required in the field to validate this belief.

The main issue raised in this chapter is the fact that our bodies are constantly under siege by thousands of poisonous agents, yet many of us remain healthy. The reason is that the healthy body is able to drain the toxins away. If this drainage system is not working properly, problems will arise and illnesses such as CFS/ME will occur.

The case of Mr F

Age: 29 years
Occupation: Designer
Marital status: Living with girlfriend, no children.

Mr F spends most of his time at work, bent over a draughtboard. His hobbies include walking and cycling. He first complained of pain in his upper and mid-dorsal spine two and a half years before first attending my practice. This pain was accompanied by dizziness, headaches and 'muzziness' in his head. (I have noticed that this muzzy feeling is a frequent symptom of CFS/ME, and is described as 'a feeling that the head is disjointed from the rest of the body', or that patient's thought processes seem to be in a permanent fog.)

Eight years prior to the onset of what turned out to be CFS/ME, Mr F had been involved in a car crash in which he was knocked unconscious and suffered concussion. He also sustained a whiplash injury of the neck and received osteopathy at the time, which relieved his neck pain.

When he first mentioned the accident, I immediately thought of blaming all his symptoms on the concussion and whiplash. It was, after all, plausible that the mechanical strain to the cervical spine had resulted in increased muscle tone in the head and neck. However, the muzziness and the fact that the symptoms worsened after any activity led me to suspect that CFS/ME was the cause of his existing complaint.

His GP had diagnosed depression and had already prescribed antidepressants, an obvious source of toxicity. Since he had been helped by osteopathy before, Mr F decided to see if manipulation would once again alleviate his symptoms. With mechanical treatment and gentle mobility exercises, his symptoms improved. The therapy began with weekly sessions, which were spread out as his health got better. After about a year he was able to carry out many more activities without any bad reaction.

Thereafter he attended for periodic check-ups and, after busy periods at work, with stress, his symptoms did return, and this I found was directly connected to the state of his upper back. Once I increased the mobility in his upper dorsal spine and relaxed the muscles of his neck, shoulder and back, he immediately felt improved. The problem was that the position he adopted at work was not the best posture for a CFS/ME sufferer. Still, with the exercise I prescribed and the occasional session of osteopathy, his quality of life drastically improved. When he was eventually discharged, he was a far more relaxed and happy man, with no need for antidepressant medication.

This case illustrates why CFS/ME used to be termed Yuppie Flu. Mr F is in what many would class as a 'young, upwardly mobile' type of job. People who spend long periods at a desk or draughtboard are putting a strain on the upper region of their back, at the principal area of spinal sympathetic activity. This factor, coupled with the stressful conditions of high profile jobs, may account for the frequent occurrence of CFS/ME in young, upwardly mobile men and women.

Chapter 8

The stages leading to CFS/ME

> All truth passes through three stages. First, it is ridiculed. Second, it is violently opposed. Third, it is accepted as being self-evident.
>
> *Arthur Schopenhauer (1788–1860)*

To treat CFS/ME successfully one has to understand the exact nature of the disease and what is going wrong with the body. Once one comprehends the stages (see Table 1 on page 77) that lead to CFS/ME, one can start to correct the disturbances, otherwise the treatment will remain only palliative rather than curative.

Three predominant concepts surfaced from the clinical trials on CFS/ME patients carried out during my eleven years of research at the universities of Salford and Manchester.

The clinical trials 1994–2005

I embarked on my clinical research in 1989 following the success of my work with the cyclist, Mr E, mentioned at the start of Chapter 1. My first paper was published in the *British Osteopathic Journal* in 1993.[1] The husband of one of my patients was a professor at the University of Salford, a large university in the Greater Manchester region with a major health sciences faculty. He showed my paper to his good friend, Professor Jack Edwards, a world-renowned bio-engineer. Professor Edwards invited me to lunch with psychology Reader, Dr Pat Hartley. Over the next three years we conducted the first clinical trial, which eventually led to the paper: 'An evaluation of the effectiveness of osteopathic treatment on symptoms associated with Myalgic

Encephalomyelitis. A preliminary report', published in the *Journal of Medical Engineering and Technology* in 1998.[2]

Hardly any research into CFS/ME was being funded by grant bodies in the 1990s, and most of the research trusts that were offering funding stipulated that it had to be paid into another charitable trust. Consequently, the Fund for Osteopathic Research into ME (FORME) was born on 23 February 1995 at The Midland Hotel, Manchester. The FORME trust was set up together with a group of my patients and friends to help raise research funds and awareness of the physical nature of CFS/ME. Thanks to donations from grateful patients, and from interested members of the public, together with donations from other trusts, we raised around £250,000 to fund the entire project.

Once you have the funding and the volunteers for a clinical trial, you need official approval from the local health authority research ethics committee. This is even more rigorous than a congressional hearing, with a group of health authority administrators, doctors, scientists and legal representatives. We encountered many complex obstacles, but eventually, by changing the protocol a number of times and by satisfying every question, we were able to start the research projects. Research ethics committees are without doubt necessary (established following the horrors of the experiments conducted by the Nazis during World War II), but one wonders how many research projects, which could improve our knowledge and treatment of disease, do not go ahead due to the exhaustive and detailed process of obtaining the necessary approval.

The efficacy of my manual approach was tested using **two separate clinical trials**, both with groups matched for gender and age. In the first trial we recruited 40 CFS/ME patients who were to be treated using my technique and 40 CFS/ME patients who were given the treatment of their choice. The second trial was a smaller study using three groups of nine subjects each. The first group consisted of CFS/ME patients who received the Perrin technique. The second group was made up of CFS/ME patients who did not receive my treatment, with the third comprised of nine healthy volunteers. This research was carried out at the universities of Salford and Manchester between 1994 and 2005 under the guidance of bioengineer Professsor Jim Richards, neurobiologist Dr Vic Pentreath and neuro-radiologist Professor Alan Jackson:

1. The first study examined the change in symptoms following a year of treatment.
2. The second study repeated the first study and examined the possible mechanisms of any improvement.

The studies were designed to develop a greater understanding of the cause, diagnosis and treatment of CFS/ME, around which much scientific uncertainty exists. Phase 1 of the research trials examined overall symptom change. It included the patient completing a selection of self-report questionnaires which were answered periodically over the course of the year-long treatment. These eight questionnaires related to feelings of depression, anxiety, cognitive function, sleep and overall health. With post-exercise fatigue being a major symptom of CFS/ME, we tested the effects of the treatment by the amount of power the quadriceps muscle in the thigh lost after a specific isometrc exercise in which the subject pushed their right shin against a pressure pad with no actual movement of the leg. The pad was connected to a gauge that measured force.

The second trial, which included the same self-reporting questionnaires assessing symptom change as the initial trial, was divided into two parallel phases, phases 2 and 3. Phase 2 primarily took the form of brain analysis using magnetic resonance imaging (MRI) to confirm if brain abnormalities seen in previous research[3,4,5] were found in sufferers of CFS/ME. Central lymph scans were also carried out to see if there was any possible enlargement in the thoracic duct of CFS/ME sufferers. In phase 3, isometric tests were carried out as in phase 1 but with much more accurate computerised equipment.[6]

The precise objectives of this research were:

1. To determine whether or not spinal problems were related to the signs and symptoms arising from CFS/ME.
2. To test if my method of osteopathic treatment reduced symptoms associated with CFS/ME compared with those of a matched control group, who received no such treatment.
3. To reveal the sustainability of any improvement by a one-year follow-up study and to investigate the likely replication of the initial study, thus strengthening the argument of a relationship between set osteopathic procedures and the improvement in signs and symptoms associated with CFS/ME.
4. To determine if there is a visible disease process in the brain that may be causing the symptoms of CFS/ME.
5. To determine if there is any intrinsic muscle disorder that may be causing the symptoms of fatigue in CFS/ME.

Conclusions of the research

I. The first stage of the research showed that the major signs and symptoms associated with CFS/ME showed an average of 40 per cent improvement in the treated group compared with an average worsening of 1 per cent in the untreated group. Muscle fatigue was shown to be significantly reduced in the treated group compared with little change in the untreated patients.

II. In the second stage of the trials it was concluded that muscle fatigue is of a functional nature rather than resulting from any known muscle disease. Secondly, following scanning the brain with magnetic resonance imaging (MRI) to examine the white matter, blood flow and cerebrospinal fluid flow, we discovered that in the CFS/ME patients there was no detectable pathological structural abnormality in the brain. (This contradicts other studies that have shown brain anomalies.[3,4,5] This conundrum may be explained by there being severe cases of CFS/ME in which the brain structure is damaged. However, our research showed that even though a person may have CFS/ME, it does not mean, necessarily, that any damage will be visible on scans. The fact that no major physical abnormality was seen in any of our CFS/ME patients suggests that visible structural trauma of the brain using standard MRI scanning methods itself is uncommon rather than the norm.)

III. Thirdly, when examining the effects of the treatment programme in both clinical trials, it seems likely that the improvement in the muscular fatigue together with the overall reduction in all CFS/ME symptoms was a result of increasing toxic drainage from the central nervous system.

The downward spiral

With careful consideration of the clinical findings, I have formulated a theoretical model to explain the cause, signs and symptoms of CFS/ME and the effectiveness of my treatment regime. My belief is the osteopathic approach does not set out directly to eliminate poisons from the body; rather, it facilitates the patient's own inbuilt mechanisms responsible for toxin elimination. By reducing the intensity of incoming sympathetic impulses, by means of relaxing the muscles and improving circulation and drainage, the signs and symptoms of CFS/ME are diminished.

My theoretical model of the stages of development of CFS/ME (see Table 1, page 77) may be applied to all the CFS/ME patients I have seen since the late 1980s.

Table 1 The stages of development of CFS/ME

Stage 1	Patients with CFS/ME all seem to have a predisposing history of sympathetic nervous system overload: a. Physically – by being an overachiever at work, during study, or in sports. Rarely, it may be the opposite by being too sedentary. b. Chemically – by constant exposure to environmental pollution. c. Immunologically – by chronic infections or hypersensitivities to multiple allergens. d. Psychologically/emotionally – by family and/or work related mental stress.
Stage 2	In Stage 2 either Stage 2a or Stage 2b can occur before the other or they can occur concurrently, depending on the causes of the restricted flow of lymphatic drainage in the head and spine.
Stage 2a	Lymphatic drainage of the central nervous system shows signs of being impaired, mostly in the cribriform plate region of the ethmoid bone above the nasal passages.
Stage 2b	Lymphatic drainage of the central nervous system is subject to disturbance in the spine, usually in the cervical or thoracic region, due to either a congenital, hereditary, or postural defect and/or prior trauma.
Stage 3	Toxic effects due to the long-term dysfunction of the central nervous system drainage will compound the chronic hyperactivity of the sympathetic nervous system; this further overloads the hypothalamus and subsequently, the sympathetic nervous system.
Stage 4	A final trigger factor strikes, which usually arises from a viral infection, but may be physical or emotional in nature.
Stage 5	There will be a disturbance in autonomic, as well as hormonal, function, because toxins in the cerebral blood flow and ventricular system directly affect control of the hypothalamus. Hormonal transport within the cerebrospinal fluid may be directly affected by toxic overload.
Stage 6	Dysfunction of sympathetic control of the thoracic duct leads to a reflux of toxins in the resultant retrograde lymph flow, causing varicose lymphatic vessels predominantly in the abdomen, neck and chest. This further reduces flow of cerebrospinal fluid into the lymphatics.
Stage 7	Further impairment of toxic drainage of the central nervous system, due to the retrograde lymphatics, results in increased hypothalamic dysfunction and an even greater reduction of lymphatic drainage.
Stage 8	The continuing irritation of the sympathetic nervous system results in further systemic disturbances, leading to a chronic adaptive state known as CFS/ME.

The physical signs of CFS/ME

The concept of CFS/ME being primarily a physical rather than psychological disorder is foreign to most of the medical profession. However, many doctors recognise that CFS/ME causes physical signs and symptoms.[7–10] There are physical components within the internationally recognised criteria that verify the diagnosis of CFS/ME.[8] These include sore throat, tender lymph nodes in the neck and armpits, and muscle and joint pain. In the seventeen years since I started to examine and treat patients with CFS/ME, repeated patterns of physical signs have emerged among all the sufferers that cannot be dismissed as pure coincidence. All physical phenomena seen in CFS/ME can be understood when the disease is viewed as the consequence of impaired drainage of the central nervous system, resulting in dysfunction of the sympathetic nervous system. The main physical signs are shown below.

1a Varicose lymphatics
1b Perrin's point
2 Coeliac plexus tenderness
3 Longstanding thoracic spinal problem, with tenderness at T4/T5/T6 segments
4 Reduction in regular sacro-cranial rhythym

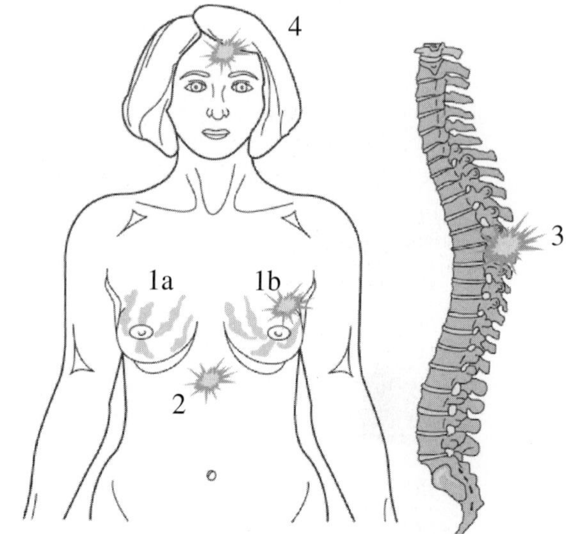

Figure 9. *The observed physical signs of CFS/ME.*
These regions of tenderness or dysfunction have been identified in all CFS/ME sufferers seen by the author since 1989 in both the university and clinical settings.

Varicose lymphatics and Perrin's Point

In every CFS/ME patient, whether male or female, there was a very tender area in the upper lateral region of the breast tissue, roughly 2 cm superior and lateral to the left nipple (Figs 9 and 10). This is the area where the pectoral muscles and lymphatic tissue overlap. This finding is significant because the tender area almost always lies on the left side and is level with the position at which the thoracic duct turns to the left. The heart and the main blood vessels are supplied with sympathetic nerves via a bundle of nerves called the cardiac plexus, which has a greater concentration of nerves on the left than the right. Sympathetic nerves run alongside the larger nerves that control movement and sensation in the body (the somatic nerves). There are often impulses crossing over from sympathetic nerves to somatic and vice versa.[11] When the cardiac rhythm is affected in CFS/ME the sympathetic nerves send messages to the sensory nerves on the left side of the chest. The thoracic duct travels from the right side to the left side of body above the level of the nipple and so, sympathetic nerves controlling the thoracic duct's pumping action are more left-sided. Thus, when these nerves are irritated, they also disturb the adjacent sensory nerves. The resultant pain is at the confluence of these two sets of sensory nerves: I refer to this tender spot as Perrin's Point.

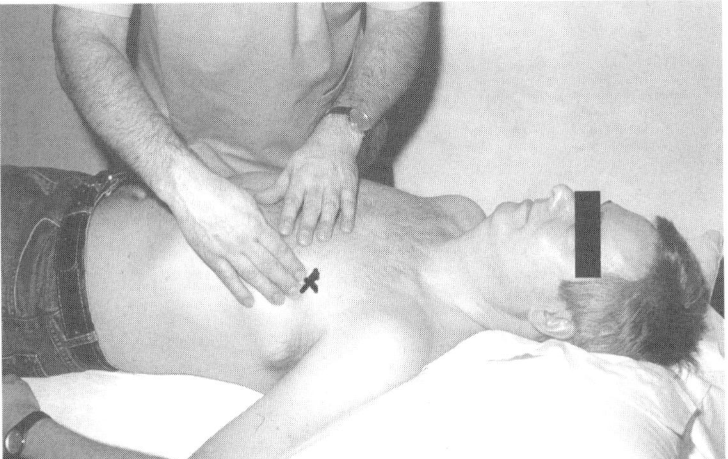

Figure 10. *Examining the patient for 'Perrin's point'.*
Gentle pressure at a point slightly superior and lateral to the left nipple "Perrin's Point"(**X**). The amount of sensitivity at this point appears to correspond to the severity of lymphatic engorgement in the breast tissue and also seems to mirror the gravity of the other symptoms.

The sensitive region, Perrin's Point, together with congested lymph vessels in the cervical region and breast tissue, was palpated (felt) in the 40 patients chosen for my treatment in the first trial and all of the 18 CFS/ME patients in the second phase of the study. The consistency of these lymphatics can best be described as 'beady' and similar to varicose veins in the leg. Varicosities (see below) have been described in the lymphatic system.[12,13,14] Large incompetent varicose lymphatic, known as megalymphatics, have often been seen when there is a back-flow of fluid within the lymphatic vessels, due to a disturbance of the normal pumping mechanism. However, varicosities in the lymphatics are rarely discussed in clinics, due to the misconception that lymph flow can only be unidirectional due to the valvular system in the lymphatic vessels. Sluggish lymph flow is known to exist in many disease states[15] and is treated by many practitioners world-wide trained in manual lymphatic drainage. However, the concept of a reverse pump causing an actual back-flow is not generally recognised clinically. Thus the possibility of a varicose lymph vessel is rarely considered when a GP or hospital consultant conducts an examination.

Downward pressure due to thoracic duct pump dysfunction caused by sympathetic disequilibrium may lead to a contra-flow within the lymphatics,[16] damaging the valves and creating a pooling of lymphatic fluid with 'beading' of the vessels. Stasis (fluid not moving) in these varicose lymphatic vessels creates risk of toxic overload together with additional damage to the lymphatics and surrounding tissue. Reflux of toxins via lymphatic vessels back into the cerebrospinal fluid will further irritate the central nervous system. Increased toxicity within the central nervous system continues to overload the sympathetic nerves, resulting in a downward spiral of deteriorating health.

From the earliest days of osteopathy, the importance of good lymphatic drainage in the thoracic duct has been seen as paramount to sustain health.[17–20] It was emphasised that, together with good blood supply, it was equally important to have perfect drainage. This is the pathway I believe to be compromised mechanically as part of the root of CFS/ME. Mechanical dysfunction such as this can be detected by palpation and can be released by gentle pressure and massage techniques applied to the cranium and the spine and surrounding soft tissue.

The healthy lymphatic vessel allows only unidirectional flow due to the valvular system as illustrated in Fig. 11. In CFS/ME, retrograde flow of the lymphatics is produced by the reverse peristaltic wave of the thoracic duct that arises from dysfunctional sympathetic control of the duct's smooth muscle wall (see Fig. 12). Eventually, the lymphatic reflux causes damage to the valves and allows pooling of fluid in between the valves. This leads to distension of the vessel wall with the characteristic beaded appearance of a varicose vessel as illustrated in Fig. 13.

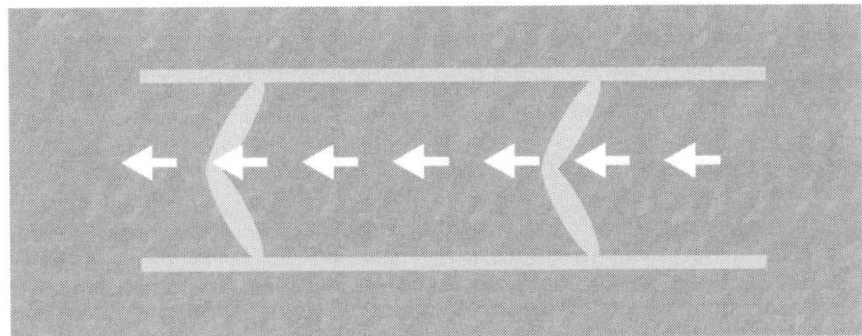

Figure 11. *Schematic illustration showing normal flow within a healthy lymphatic vessel.* The valves in this healthy vessel are intact preventing any backflow, thus maintaining a unidirectional flow of lymphatic fluid.

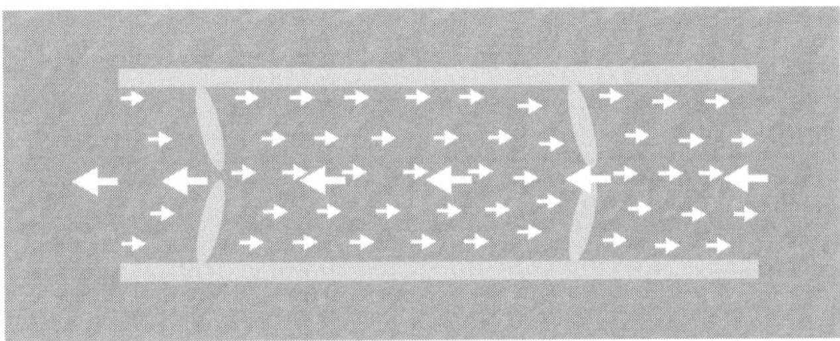

Figure 12. *Schematic illustration showing retrograde lymphatic flow.*
If the normal peristaltic wave of the thoracic duct is disturbed resulting in reflux, then the ensuing back-pressure will weaken the valves allowing a retrograde flow.

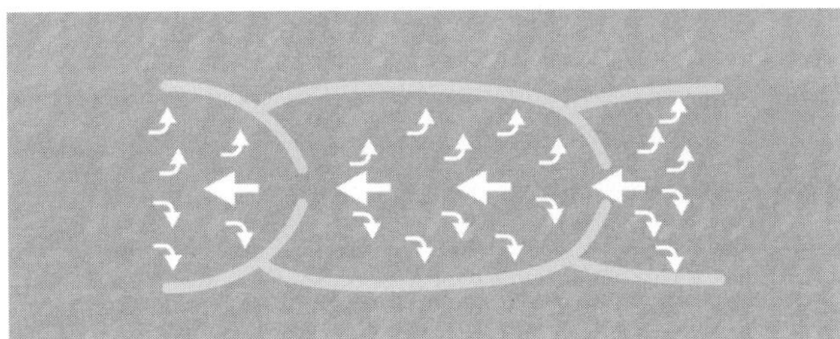

Figure 13. *Schematic illustration showing the formation of lymphatic varicosities.*
The walls between the collapsed valves become noticeably distended with further reflux of lymphatic fluid.

Fig. 14 shows the top right section of the chest of a 61 year old man. One can see the swollen, tortuous beaded vessels just beneath the collar bone adjacent to the right shoulder. The man suffered severely from CFS/ME for four years before being successfully treated with a two-year course of osteopathy. The beaded appearance in Fig. 14 is due to damaged valves and subsequent retrograde flow and pooling of lymphatic fluid. This is similar to the formation of varicose veins, although it lacks the darker, bluish hue of superficial varicose veins. The creamy appearance of lymph is almost apparent in these engorged vessels, which have a much larger diameter than in normal healthy superficial lymphatic vessels. It is extremely rare to see such pronounced superficial varicose megalymphatics as illustrated here. However, I have been able to feel the presence of varicose lymphatic vessels in the neck and chest of all the CFS/ME patients I have seen since 1989.

Tenderness at solar plexus

The largest major autonomic plexus, uniting two large coeliac ganglia, is known as the **coeliac plexus**, more commonly referred to as the solar plexus. This major confluence of nerves is level with the 12th thoracic/1st lumbar segment and is situated posterior to the stomach and in front of tendonous insertions of the diaphragm. Secondary plexuses connected to the coeliac plexus are: phrenic; splenic; hepatic; left gastric; intermesenteric; suprarenal; renal; testicular/ovarian;

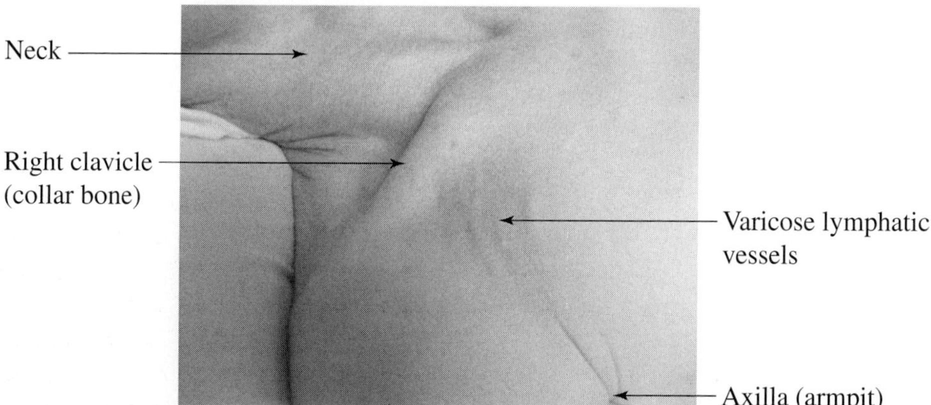

Figure 14. *Right subclavicular varicose lymphatics in patient with CFS/ME.*
Four years after completing a 2 year treatment programme, one can clearly see five separate varicose lymphatic vessels under the skin at the anterior medial aspect of the right shoulder, the central one being the most pronounced. (See plate I, opposite.)

Plate I

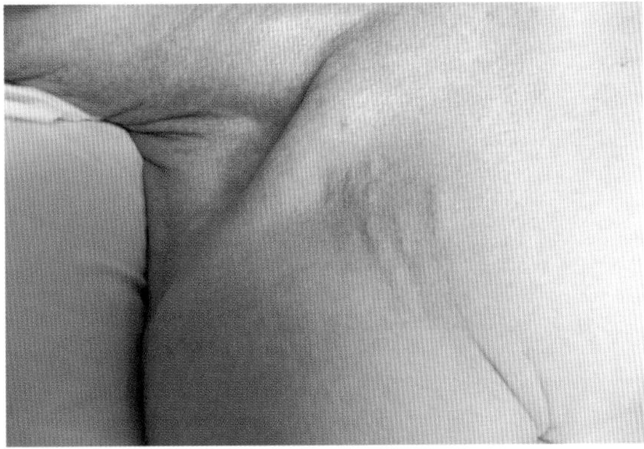

Right subclavicular varicose lymphatics in patient with CFS/ME.
Four years after completing a 2 year treatment programme, one can clearly see five separate varicose lymphatic vessels under the skin at the anterior medial aspect of the right shoulder, the central one being the most pronounced.

superior and inferior mesenteric, sending and receiving messages from all the abdominal organs and below.

Through its connections, the solar plexus is excellent as an indicator for any visceral disturbances from the waist down. Tenderness in this abdominal region, known as the epigastrium, seems to be directly related to the severity of any lower extremity fatigue and/or abdominal problem. This is due to impulses passing across the connections between adjacent sensory and sympathetic nerves.

Postural/structural dysfunction of the thoracic spine

A prevailing observation in the clinical findings of CFS/ME is a mechanical disorder of the thoracic spine, which may be due to bad occupational posture, or related to a congenital event or genetic predisposition. All of the patients in the studies that I undertook had a particular dysfunction in the thoracic region, whether it was inflammation, abnormal curvature, or just a restricted area.

A common structural disturbance seen by myself in CFS/ME patients was a flattening of the curvature in the mid-thoracic spine, usually accompanied by the presence of a kyphotic dorso-lumbar area (an abnormally exaggerated convex curvature in the lower back). An example of this defect is shown in Fig. 15a which

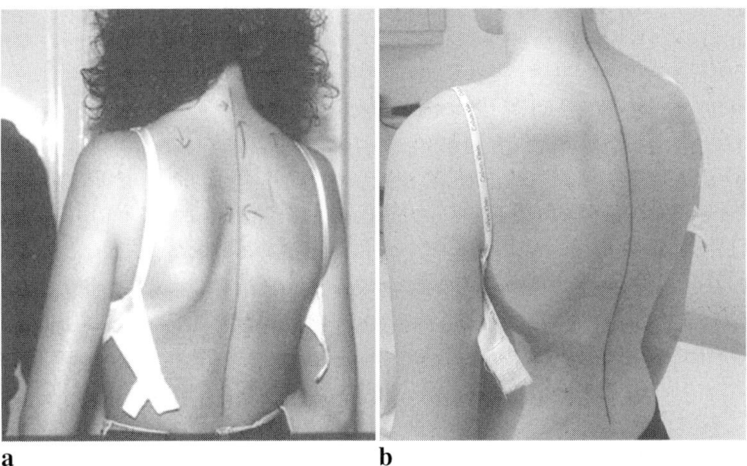

a **b**

Figure 15. *Comparative photographs showing a flattened mid-thoracic spine.*
Photo **a** on the left shows the familiar flattening of the mid thoracic spine seen in many CFS/ME patients. This differs from a normal spinal posture in the healthy subject on the right, **b**.

can be compared with the healthy posture shown in Fig. 15b. This postural defect is often caused by a prior condition, osteochondrosis, also known as Scheurmann's disease, which affects spinal development in adolescence and which may have occurred years before the onset of the characteristic symptoms of CFS/ME.

Changes in cranio-sacral rhythm

There is a palpable rhythmic pulsation along the spinal cord and around the brain together with that of normal breathing, which is transmitted to the rest of the body and is termed the 'involuntary mechanism', 'cranial rhythmic impulse' (CRI), or the 'cranio-sacral rhythm'. Most of the osteopathic profession believe the pulse to be a movement through the tension and continuity of membranes and fascia. The fascia consists of connective tissue that is continuous with the membranes that surround the brain and spinal cord, the meninges, thus allowing any motion within the nervous system to be transmitted throughout the body.

William Garner Sutherland (1873–1954), the founder of cranial osteopathy, proposed that there was a primary respiratory mechanism created within the central nervous system via the spinal cord; he believed that the bones in the cranium all moved in a rhythmic pattern together with the sacrum at the base of the spine.[19]

Sutherland proposed that the primary respiratory mechanism produces a rhythmic alternation of flexion and extension of structures in the midline. This movement occurs simultaneously with the rhythmic external and internal rotation of all paired lateral structures such as the kidneys.

It has been suggested that contractile lymph tissue exists throughout the body, which creates a powerful pumping mechanism.[12] It has been shown that the thoracic duct pump influences the drainage of cerebrospinal fluid/lymph from the central nervous system. Together with the pulse rate and the effects of breathing, a separate underlying rhythm may be induced; this may be the aforementioned 'involuntary mechanism'[21]. This rhythm echoes along the lymphatic system, resonating throughout the entire body and can be palpated by trained practitioners. In CFS/ME patients it is slow and its intensity shallower than in healthy subjects. I found this to be the case in all the CFS/ME patients that I examined clinically and during my research.

Conclusion

Recognition of the diagnostic signs that I have described (see Fig 9) can be taught, easily, to clinicians. There are plenty of practitioners trained in cranio-sacral techniques who can apply all the diagnostic procedures, described above, that may identify CFS/ME in its earliest stages. In fact, when examining siblings or children of CFS/ME patients, I have discovered that the physical signs often appear long before the symptoms present themselves fully. It is possible in such familial cases to diagnose a pre-CFS/ME condition and prevent individuals from succumbing to the full-blown illness. I believe that I am the only practitioner to claim that CFS/ME is preventable (see Chapter 11). One thing is certain: the earlier that a patient receives a definite diagnosis, and thus the correct treatment, the better are the chances of that person's recovery.

The case of Mrs H

Age: 21 years
Occupation: Housewife
Marital status: Married for one year.

Mrs H's symptoms began with abdominal pains and she had already been diagnosed with irritable bowel syndrome (IBS) when she first came to see me. This common disorder is thought to be due either to abnormal motility within the gut or a heightened sensitivity to distension of the intestine. In Mrs H's case, the abdominal cramps were accompanied by aches in the limbs and dizziness, and she had felt lethargic for a few years. These symptoms are not usually associated with IBS, and she came to me feeling quite depressed.

When she first consulted me, she was a few weeks' pregnant. She had informed me about a miscarriage which had occurred a few months earlier. The news of her pregnancy came just before I was to advise her of the need to use a contraceptive device until her symptoms had improved.

There are two viewpoints concerning pregnancy and CFS/ME. Some experts believe that pregnancy is a time when a better balance is achieved within the woman's body and it can help reduce the symptoms of CFS/ME. However, this is unpredictable. Some healthy women blossom when pregnant: if the CFS/ME patient is lucky enough to be that type, her symptoms will probably reduce during pregnancy. However, if the mother-to be is one of those who generally have a difficult pregnancy, her CFS/ME symptoms may worsen for most of the nine months as her hormonal levels fluctuate, producing more nausea and fatigue.

The increase in weight and the changes in overall posture of the mother-to-be put much more mechanical strain on her back. From a mechanical point of view, some women may feel more mobility in the spine during pregnancy. This is due to the hormone relaxin, which is released from the ovaries throughout pregnancy. This hormone, as its name suggests, causes joints and ligaments to loosen. The relaxation of the joints prepares the body for the mechanical pressure put on the spine and pelvis during the later stages of pregnancy and, eventually, labour. The effects of the hormone lead to many pregnant women suffering from strained joints, for example, sprained ankles. However, the consequent increase in movement in the thoracic and upper spine may be beneficial in CFS/ME sufferers.

Mrs H's upper dorsal spine was severely restricted. This stiffness probably dated back to an accident when she was only 15 years old, in which she had fallen badly and injured her head. Since then, she had suffered bouts of depression and had been prescribed antidepressants, which gave no relief. An antispasmodic pill was also prescribed for the abdominal cramps with no success.

With regular treatment throughout her pregnancy, I was able to maintain some mobility in her upper spine, and her general condition improved slightly. The most encouraging factor was that her symptoms did not worsen. In the latter months, with the help of relaxin, the mobility in her spine greatly increased and she noted how well she felt during the last few weeks of pregnancy.

I advised her to deliver the baby on her side. The left-lateral position is commonly used when patients have spinal problems. Lying on the back in the standard position of delivery puts enormous strain on the spine, and this would have caused a worsening of her symptoms after the birth.

She eventually gave birth to a healthy 8 lb (3.6 kg) baby girl. There were no complications during labour and a few weeks after the birth, when Mrs H came for a check-up, she was feeling much healthier and more energetic. She coped extremely well with her new baby and the aches and pains were no longer a problem.

Chapter 9

Osteopathy

> It is a perfectly well established technique, there is no mystery about it. It ought to be part of the equipment of every doctor in the country.
>
> *George Bernard Shaw (1856–1950), speaking about osteopathy in 1927*

Many of you reading this book may be more familiar with CFS/ME than with osteopathy and you may by now have a clearer understanding of the mechanical processes leading to CFS/ME, but still you may be wondering how osteopathy can help.

Osteopathic treatment

Current treatment for CFS/ME includes dietary regimes, with evidence to suggest that essential fatty acid intake must be normalised in the management of the disease. Psychotherapy, exercise programmes and antidepressants have all been advocated. The different treatment programmes all – whether chemical, hormonal, or psychological – focus on palliative treatment rather than cure.

Osteopaths aim to treat CFS/ME by reducing the irritation of the sympathetic nervous system in the patient, thus allowing a return to a healthy homeostatic state. My hypothesis is that this can be achieved by increasing the drainage of toxins from the cerebrospinal fluid via the lymphatics. The treatment also reduces the tone of the sympathetic nervous system by improving the structure and overall quality of movement of the lower cervical, dorsal and upper lumbar regions of the spine, together with relaxation of the surrounding musculature.

The two sympathetic trunks (see page 25) are integrally related to the overall structure of this area. By reducing mechanical irritation, disturbed sympathetic afferent impulses may be minimised, further helping to stabilise blood and lymph flow. My core theory proposes that the breakdown of this system is central to the disease process of CFS/ME and that, by restoring the neurological equilibrium, one reduces the metabolic disturbance, thus addressing the cause of the symptoms.

History and principles of osteopathy

"Osteopathy is the knowledge of the structure, relations and functions of each part and tissue of the human body applied to the adjustment and correction of whatever may be interfering with their harmonious operation," to quote A.T. Still.[1]

Dr Andrew Taylor Still (1828–1917) of Kirksville, Missouri, founded osteopathy in the latter part of the nineteenth century as an alternative to the poor quality of medicine practised at the time. He called his new system of medicine 'osteopathy' from the Greek words for bone *osteon* and disease *pathos*. His basic tenet for viewing the body as a machine was based upon his religious beliefs and upon his despair at the futility of most medication available at the time. He formulated his original hypothesis from Biblical text. 'Let Us make man in Our image,' *Genesis* Ch 1, verse 26. Still, who was the son of a minister, took this verse literally. He postulated that if The Creator is perfect, man must have been made perfect. As he stated, "The principles of osteopathy give us an understanding of the perfect plans and specifications followed in man's construction". Osteopathy teaches that structure governs function. Thus illness, Still maintained, develops when the perfect structure is out of balance.

Osteopathy became popular in the American mid-west and there are now twenty established osteopathic medical schools in the USA, with an enrolment of nearly 10,000 students. The first osteopathic college in the UK was The British School of Osteopathy, established in 1921. Today, there are over 3,000 osteopaths in the UK registered with the General Osteopathic Council, formed by Act of Parliament in 1998. The profession is now accepted in Great Britain, to some extent, with other mainstream medical disciplines.

According to the General Osteopathic Council, osteopathy is an established recognised system of diagnosis and treatment, which lays its main emphasis on the structural and functional integrity of the body. It is distinguished by the fact that it recognises that much of the pain and disability we suffer stems from abnormalities in the structure of the body and their effects on function as well as damage caused by disease.

How osteopathy helps

One of the major concepts of osteopathy is that the structure of the body governs the function of the organs within. Osteopaths work on the principle that a patient's history of illnesses and physical traumas are written into the body's structure. It is the osteopath's developed palpatory sense that enables the practitioner manually to diagnose while treating the patient. The osteopath's job is to restore a healthy structure to the body and thus restore its function. The osteopath gently applies manual techniques of massage and manipulation to encourage movement of body fluids, eliminate dysfunction in the motion of the tissues, relax muscular tension and release compressed bones and joints. The areas being treated require proper positioning to assist the body's ability to regain normal tissue function.

One of Still's students, William Sutherland, noticed that when the bones of a disarticulated skull were viewed in a certain way, they resembled the gills of a fish. Accordingly, he hypothesised in 1898, that their shape was designed to allow for movement and, as explained in Chapter 8, cranial osteopathy was born.[2]

Drainage of toxins

The main lymphatic vessels are known to be under the control of the sympathetic nervous system. The smooth muscle wall of the thoracic duct, when stimulated, produces a wave of contraction – peristalsis – aiding lymph drainage into the subclavian vein. This produces a negative pressure along the lymphatics and aids further lymph drainage.

The choroid plexus in the brain consists of many blood capillaries which allow fluid to filter out, becoming cerebrospinal fluid. Sutherland emphasised the importance of the choroid plexus in the chemical exchange between cerebrospinal fluid and the blood (see Fig 1, page 5), but stressed the part played by the lymphatics in the drainage of toxins from the central nervous system. He said, 'When you tap the waters of the brain by compressing the fourth ventricle see what happens in the lymphatic system. Visualise the lymph node that is holding some poison that has gathered there, changing the constituency before the lymph is moved along into the venous system."[2]

Andrew Taylor Still discussed the importance of examining disturbed fluid motion in the head, in the pathogenesis of many signs and symptoms such as headaches, enlarged tonsils, dizziness and loss of memory, all associated with CFS/ME. 'We strike at the source of life and death when we go into the lymphatics.'[3] Still emphasised that it was equally important to have perfect drainage as well as good blood supply.

This includes drainage of mucus from our noses. Sutherland postulated that each of the sinuses behind the face has one or more bones that help drain mucus, which is produced in special cells called 'goblet' cells that line the inside (epithelium) of the sinuses, by a gentle pumping action. This facilitates a wafting action that forces the mucus into the nasopharynx (back of the throat). When mechanical or other forces damage this mechanism, the sinus is less able to drain the mucus. As a result, the mucus pools, thickens and makes us prone to infection. The nasal mucosa may then become continually inflamed with large amounts of purulent mucus and associated enlargement of our adenoids and tonsils. Mechanical dysfunction such as this can be detected by palpation and can be released by gentle pressure techniques applied to the cranium and the spine.

Lymphatic vessels in the submucosa of the nasal sinuses are the initial recipients of the drainage of cerebrospinal fluid through the cribriform plate. As early as the1890s, Taylor Still noted, 'The lymphatics are closely and universally connected with the spinal cord and all other nerves, and all drink from the waters of the brain'.[4] From the earliest days of osteopathy the importance of good lymphatic drainage in the thoracic duct has been seen as paramount to sustain health. Taylor Still himself wrote: 'At this point I will draw your attention to what I consider is the cause of a whole list of hitherto unexplained diseases, which are only effects of the blood and other fluids being prohibited from doing normal service by constrictions at the various openings of the diaphragm. Thus prohibition of the free action of the thoracic duct would produce congestion.'[5]

The average pulsation of the cranial mechanism is believed by many practitioners to be between 8 and 12 beats per minute in health, although in some studies authorities have calculated the average rate to be 12.47 impulses per minute with the rate for normal adults being 10-14 cycles per minute(cpm).[6-9] Other investigations relying on manual palpation of the cranial rhythmic impulse (CRI) have recorded values of between 3 and 9 cpm (cycles per minute).[10-13]

At present there is no means of measuring the patient's cerebrospinal fluid's drainage into the lymphatic duct. However, clinical assessment of hundreds of CFS/ME sufferers since 1989 has revealed a weak, arrhythmic and slow CRI in patients with CFS/ME compared with any of the average healthy rates mentioned above. These findings coincided with lymphatic pump reversal leading to palpable engorged varicose lymphatics.[14, 15]

As osteopathy's founder stated over a century ago, 'Harmony only dwells where obstructions do not exist'.[16] The Perrin technique, which seeks to reduce the obstructions and restore harmony, thus has a very significant part to play in the effective treatment of people with CFS/ME.

The case of Mr I

Age: 40 years
Occupation: Computer science teacher
Marital status: Married, with one 10-year-old daughter.

When I first examined him Mr I complained of severe pain in his neck, shoulders and low back, which had been troubling him for many years. In the past, he had suffered a few minor injuries to his spine, and presented with a stiffened, arthritic thoracic spine. This postural problem was exacerbated by his profession, spending much of his working day bent over a computer console. He also complained of aches in both legs and weakness in his arms, as well as a general feeling of fatigue and dizziness. As with some of the other patients, his CFS/ME was associated with a permanent restriction of the dorsal spine due to wear and tear.

With treatment to improve the mechanics of the upper back, Mr I's symptoms of CFS/ME have improved. However, his spine will never be completely mobile, and because of the damaging nature of his work, Mr I will continue to need periodic treatment.

As soon as Mr I experiences more back pain than usual from the physical strain of his work, he immediately begins to suffer from fatigue symptoms. These are quickly relieved by manipulative treatment. The speed of his improvement following therapy neatly demonstrates the relationship between the mechanical health of the spine and CFS/ME.

Chapter 10

Treating CFS/ME

The cure for this ill is not to sit still.

Rudyard Kipling (1865–1936)

The osteopathic techniques that I have developed to treat CFS/ME patients are based on standard procedures used by trained osteopathic practitioners.[1,2] The manual treatment of each CFS/ME patient consists of a number of stages. I will describe these in some technical detail now before setting out recommendations for self-care. In particular I use a lot of anatomical terms which are necessary for precision. Non-practitioners may wish to turn immediately to 'Self-help advice' on page 103, but interested general readers can find the anatomical terms explained in a number of excellent books including *Principles of Anatomy and Physiology: the Maintenance and Continuity of the Human Body* by G. Totora *et al* (publisher, John Wiley & Sons Inc).

Stages of treatment

1. Effleurage (massage) to aid drainage in thoracic and cervical lymphatic vessels.
2. Gentle articulation of thoracic and upper lumbar spine, and the ribs. This is achieved by both long and short lever techniques.
3. Soft tissue massage of certain muscles: the paravertebral muscles, the trapezii, levator scapulae, rhomboids and muscles of respiration.

4. High and low velocity manipulation of the thoracic and upper lumbar spinal segments using supine (back-lying) and side-lying combined leverage and thrust techniques.
5. Functional techniques to the suboccipital region and the sacrum.
6. Stimulation of the cranio-sacral rhythm by functional cranial techniques.
7. Exercises are prescribed to improve the quality of thoracic spine mobility and the coordination of the patient.

The stages of treatment, as shown above, form the protocol followed throughout the clinical trials in the years 1996–7 and 2000–2001. It altered slightly, depending on the physical state of the patient and on the symptom picture at that particular stage in their therapy.

Effleurage to aid drainage in thoracic and cervical lymphatic vessels

Congested lymph and oedematous changes (swelling) are relieved by 'effleurage', a method of massage that requires stroking motions along the surface of the trunk and the neck.

The gentle strokes are carried out rhythmically towards the subclavian region, above the subclavian veins, which drain all the lymph fluid into the blood stream. Effleurage stimulates the lymphatic drainage through direct routes into the thoracic duct and hence into the venous return (see Fig. 16. page 94). Care is taken to avoid stimulating drainage into the axillary lymph nodes, which are prone to swelling and congestion in CFS/ME sufferers. It is hypothesised that the more direct route forces a high pressure within the smaller parasternal vessels, which creates enough force within the thoracic duct to alleviate the back-pressure and restore a healthy drainage of toxins into the venous return.

With female patients effleurage to the breast tissue is carried out in the presence of a chaperone, after explaining the exact nature of the treatment, and using consent forms usually supplied by the practitioner's governing body. The gentle stroking is applied upwards covering the entire breast tissue towards the clavicle (collar bone).

The effleurage technique is used on the lymphatic vessels of the neck, head and back, stroking downwards along the back and sides of the neck and head and upwards along each side of the thoracic spine. Each stroking motion finishes at the level of the subclavian vein, creating the pressure required to restore a healthy drainage of toxins.

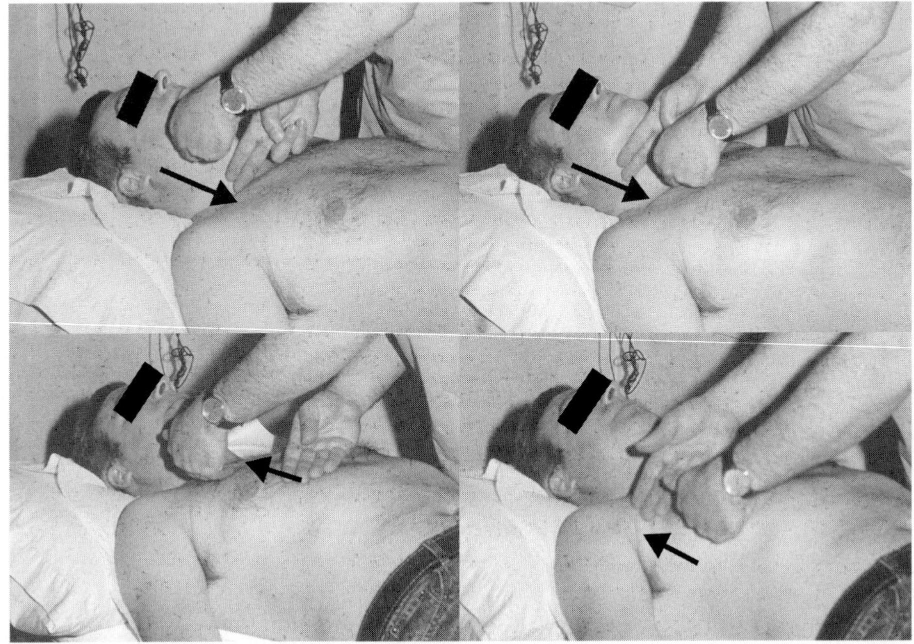

Figure 16. *Effleurage down neck and up chest to clavicle.*
The arrows show the direction of the massage technique, which is always towards either clavicle (collarbone) on both sides. This is the region above the drainage of lymphatic fluid from the right lymphatic duct and the thoracic duct into the right and left subclavian veins respectively.

Gentle articulation of thoracic and upper lumbar spine and the ribs

The main objective of the articulatory, soft tissue techniques and high velocity manipulation (stages 2, 3 and 4) is to improve the structure and overall quality of movement of the dorsal and upper lumbar spine.

The two sympathetic trunks are integrally related to the overall structure of the area. By reducing mechanical irritation at this region, as well as relaxing disturbed afferent impulses, the dysfunction of the sympathetic nervous system can be corrected.

In cases of hypermobility, which is rarely found in the patient's thoracic spine, mobility of the adjoining areas of the spine is improved by articulation and manipulation. This takes the strain off the hypermobile segments. What is predominantly found in patients with CFS/ME is a restricted dorsal spine. Frequently, the entire thoracic region is stiff, and occasionally just a few segments are affected.

Treatment to increase mobility of the spine can take many forms. The general articulatory manoeuvres employed are short lever mobilisation, using gentle pressure on the pars articularis and spinal processes, together with long lever rhythmic stretching of the dorsal and lumbar spinal segments, using the arms and legs for the appropriate leverage. All the articulatory techniques are slowly and gently applied with minimal force in order to avoid irritating spinal inflammation and to reduce any reactive spasm from the surrounding muscles.

This method is carried out with the patient lying supine (on his or her front), but mostly the patient lies on his or her side to allow a gentle stretch of periscapular and paravertebral muscles together with gentle massage upwards along the spine to improve lymphatic flow. This is often combined with a gentle stretch of the ribs, which is performed by holding the patient's arm with one hand, fixing the ribs with the other hand, and gently moving the held arm upwards, stretching the thorax above the fixed rib. Combined stretch and massage, using the patient's arm as a long-lever, produces excellent results, with movement of the ribs increased by articulatory stretch techniques (see Fig. 17).

To remedy the problems caused by hypermobile joints, as with restricted joints, the first task is to reduce any possible inflammation present at the damaged segments. This can be achieved in various ways. Some practitioners would prescribe anti-inflammatory drugs. However, contrast (hot alternating with cold) bathing is deemed preferable, as it has no toxic side effects. The hot compress usually consists of a warm (not hot) water bottle. Too hot a compress could scald the patient's skin. The 'cold' is as cold as the patient can tolerate; it is safer if a frozen pack is wrapped with a cover, especially as CFS/ME patients often cannot tolerate extremes of temperature. Frozen peas, which easily mould around the back, can be used, although special cold compress packs, which remain soft even when frozen, are more suitable.

My clinical experience has shown that the sequence of contrast bathing that gives the best results in reducing the inflammation in CFS/ME is as follows:

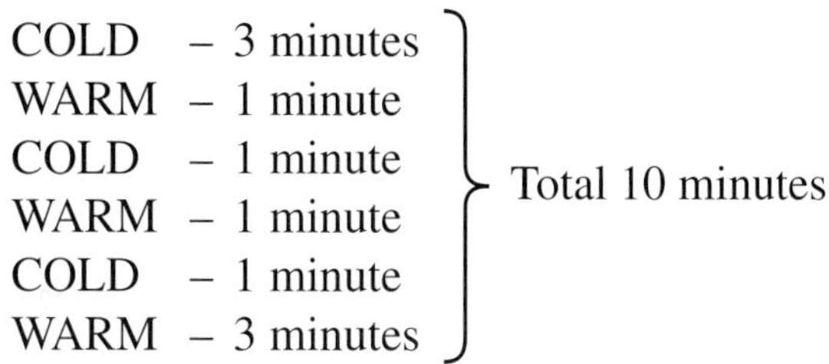

COLD – 3 minutes
WARM – 1 minute
COLD – 1 minute
WARM – 1 minute
COLD – 1 minute
WARM – 3 minutes

Total 10 minutes

This process has no adverse side-effects, and so it is safe to use as many times as required. Applications of at least three times a day to the upper thoracic region is recommended if there is inflammation in the neck and shoulders (or there are cerebral symptoms such as cognitive difficulties) and the lower thoracic area when the abdominal or lower extremities are affected. The main advantage of contrast bathing over anti-inflammatory drugs is that it works quickly and directly on the affected area. Even when there is no palpable or visible inflammation, shown by heat and redness, contrast bathing to improve circulation in the thoracic region is still advised.

Soft tissue massage of the paravertebral muscles, trapezii, levator scapulae, rhomboids and muscles of respiration

Generally, the massage technique for the relaxation of the above mentioned muscle groups takes the form of gentle longitudinal and cross-fibre stretching. Almond oil is recommended as it is the most common base oil used in massage and seems in most cases to be hypoallergenic.

With the patient lying on his or her side, paravertebral muscles, primarily the dorsal erector spinae, are manually stretched using direct longitudinal pressure up to a level parallel with the first thoracic vertebra. Combined with long lever stretching, via movement of the patient's arm and shoulder joint, this method has the added advantage of increasing rib movement and stimulating deep lymphatic drainage from the spine (see Fig. 17).

I try to avoid having the patient lie in a prone (on his or her front) position. However, if the practitioner finds it necessary for the patient to lie prone, his or her face should be placed into a breathing hole in the practice bed to avoid unnecessary strain on the neck. The patient should be moved on to the side as soon as possible to carry out the paravertebral soft tissue work in this healthier position, while keeping the head level and knees apart with the aid of pillows.

Treatment is given to relax the trapezii (see Fig. 18) and periscapular muscles, for example, the rhomboids, as well as any other hypertonic back and shoulder muscles. Besides stretching, occasionally inhibition or functional techniques are used to reduce the tone of the tightened musculature (see Fig. 22).

After increasing movement of the restricted spine and relaxing the surrounding musculature, I attempt to improve the respiratory mechanics. This is important in CFS/ME patients, since the amount of oxygen in the body affects its chemical content, and has a direct effect on the functioning of the body's tissues. Reduced oxygen produces greater fatigue in the patient and will aggravate the symptoms. By improving the mechanics of respiration in the rib cage, the patient's lung capacity is increased

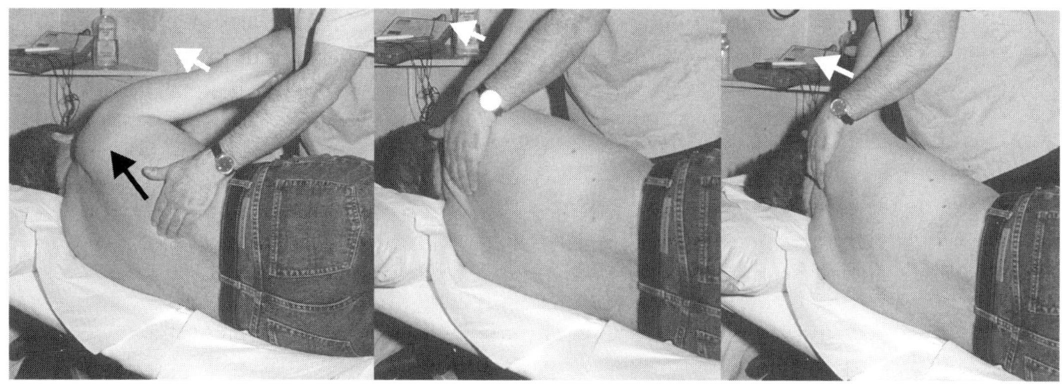

Figure 17. *Combined articulation, soft tissue stretch and paraspinal effleurage.*
This method is a combination of three soft tissue techniques: long lever stretch of the intercostals, using the patient's arm as a lever; direct longitudinal stretch of the dorsal erector spinae with the fingertips; and effleurage to the paravertebral lymphatics. The black arrow illustrates the direction of the massage and the white arrows show the direction of movement of the patient's arm.

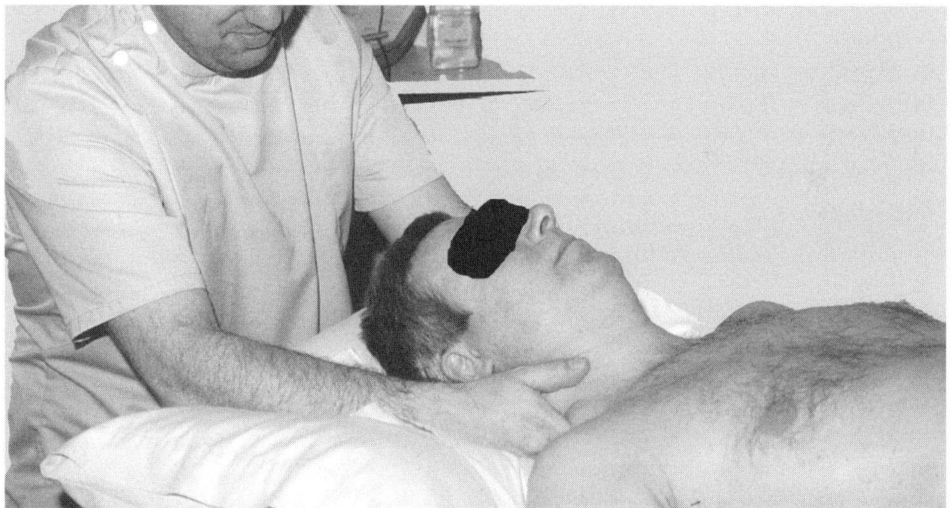

Figure 18. *Cross fibre stretching of lower neck and shoulders.*
This technique involves a slow rhythmic kneading action applied across the fibres of the lower cervical erector spinae, trapezii and levator scapulae.

during inspiration, thus raising the patient's oxygen intake. Although increasing spinal mobility and relaxing paravertebral muscles will enhance movement of the ribs, the specific respiratory muscles should also be treated in order to improve the respiratory mechanics. These include the intercostal muscles, serratus anterior and posterior, pectorals, abdominals and, most importantly, the diaphragm. Gentle inhibition to the edge of the diaphragm dome will usually reduce the tone of the muscle and aid breathing. This technique is known as 'diaphragmatic release'.

After increasing mobility of the thorax by articulation and stretching, as well as relaxing the musculature, the patient is usually feeling more comfortable and can lie in a supine position with knees slightly bent in readiness for the next stage of therapy.

High velocity-low amplitude manipulation

If any of the joints are severely immobile, it may prove necessary to increase movement by high velocity low amplitude thrust techniques (see Figs 19, 20 and 21). In osteopathy, this technique is called High Velocity-Low Amplitude (HVLA)

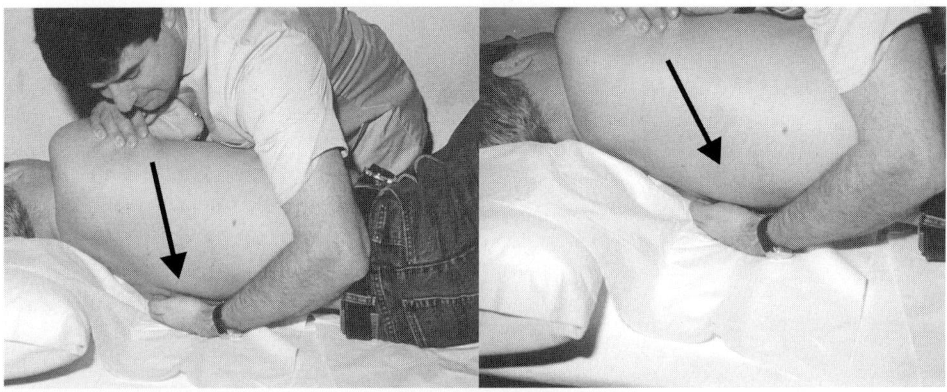

Figure 19. *Combined leverage and thrust of mid-thoracic vertebrae.*
My left hand is positioned in a loose fist around the spinous process of the vertebra. As pressure is exerted from my right hand, through the patient's body, the facet joints at the side of the adjacent vertebrae will open to *gap the facet joints*. When the tension has built up by positioning the patient's upper spine in a flexed and rotated position, a fast but gentle pressure is applied through the direction of force as illustrated by the arrow which further gaps the joint and brings about a long-lasting increase in mobility.

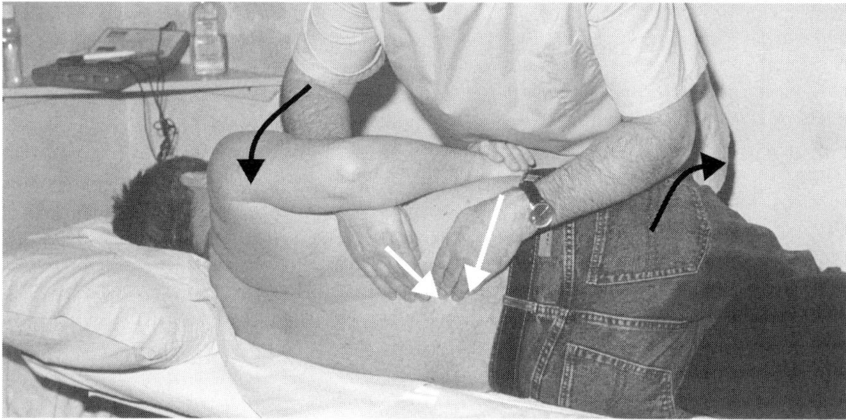

Figure 20. *Combined leverage and thrust on the upper lumbar spine.*
The upper lumbar vertebrae are gently rotated, creating a tension at a restricted joint. By applying a further quick thrust with my hands across the joint, it opens and creates more overall movement.

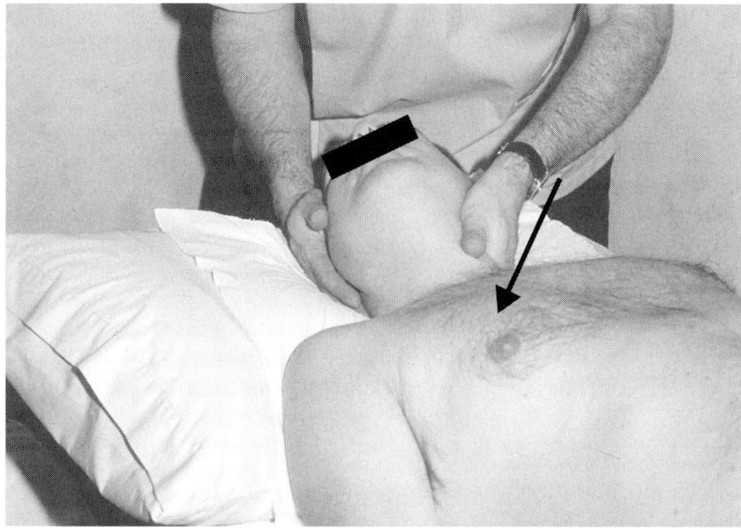

Figure 21. *Gentle combined leverage and thrust on the lower cervical spine.*
This manipulative procedure involves bending the patient's neck to the left while rotating the cervical spine towards his right. Gentle pressure is placed towards the direction of the arrow, gapping the joints at the side of the restricted vertebrae and creating more movement.

or simply the high velocity thrust (HVT). In chiropractic, this manoeuvre is called an 'adjustment' and is commonly known as a manipulation. It is the best known technique in the osteopath's armoury and involves a short, sharp motion usually applied to the spine. This procedure is designed to release structures with a restricted range of movement. There are various methods of delivering a high velocity thrust. Chiropractors are more likely to push on vertebrae with their hands, whereas osteopaths tend to use the limbs to make levered thrusts. That said, osteopathic and chiropractic techniques are converging, and much of their therapeutic repertoire is shared. This technique may produce a 'cracking' sound.

The HVTs can be achieved with the patient lying prone, but it is preferable and safer to turn the patient on to their back and manipulate them in a supine position. Vertebral joints in some patients may appear slightly fused and therefore strong manipulation should be avoided in order to prevent any damage to the bone.

The sequence, strength and duration of all the above techniques are based on each individual case, but care is taken not to over-manipulate, especially in the lower cervical region, as this can exacerbate the symptoms.

Functional techniques to the suboccipital region and the sacrum

It is important when one treats posturo-mechanical strain of the spine to balance the suboccipital and lumbosacral segments. Any abnormal curvature will alter muscular tone along the spinal column and thus place an extra load on the uppermost section and base of the spine. Similarly, positional alterations at the top and bottom of the spinal column will affect the overall mechanics of the entire spine. Osteopaths and chiropractors may use an effective procedure in these regions known as the functional technique (see Fig 22). If, during subtle movement of the spine, a restriction is detected, however slight, the back is held at the point of restriction until a release of muscle tension occurs. In practice, osteopaths rely on finely developed palpatory skills. The main principle of any osteopathic treatment is that structure governs function (see Chapter 9). The principle of the functional technique is that by placing a joint or a group of muscles in a certain position that is functionally suited for that particular bodily part, the result is a relaxation of tissues and an overall improvement in muscular and fascial tone in the region.

The suboccipital muscles and the pelvic and lower lumbar muscles can be relaxed efficiently and painlessly by gentle positioning of the occiput and sacrum respectively. With the patient lying supine, the osteopath's hands are placed at each side, cradling the occiput, which is then lifted slightly off the pillow. The cervical spine is then gently extended and slowly rotated and bent towards the right. Traction

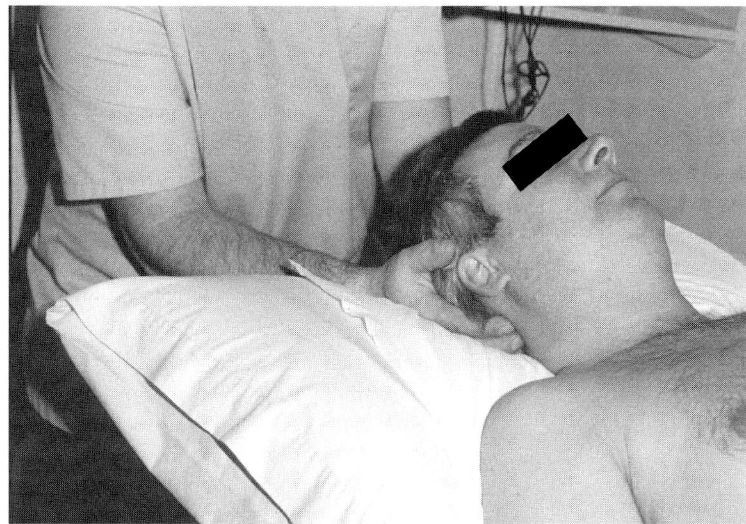

Figure 22. *Functional technique to the suboccipital region.*
With the patient lying supine, the osteopath's hands are placed at each side, cradling the occiput, which is then slightly lifted off the pillow and held in a fixed position to produce comfort and relaxation of the tissues in the upper cervical region.

or compression is applied and by asking the patient to breathe deeply, it is possible to utilise exhalation as a relaxation tool.

There is a fixed position where, by palpating the muscular tone just beneath the occiput, using the fingertips, one is able to feel the point of maximum relaxation for the suboccipital muscles. This position is held for a few seconds, resulting in a reduction of tone in this muscle group (see Fig 22).

The same technique is applied to the pelvic and lower lumbar region by cradling one hand under the patient's sacrum and palpating the muscular tone in the lumbar-sacral region.

Stimulation of the cranio-sacral rhythm

Stage six commences near the end of each consultation (see Fig 23). This useful technique is very effective at restoring energy and improving the cognitive ability of the patient.

The fluctuating slow wave previously identified by Sutherland,[3,4] and described in Chapters 8 and 9, is known as the cranial rhythmic impulse (CRI). The CRI has a

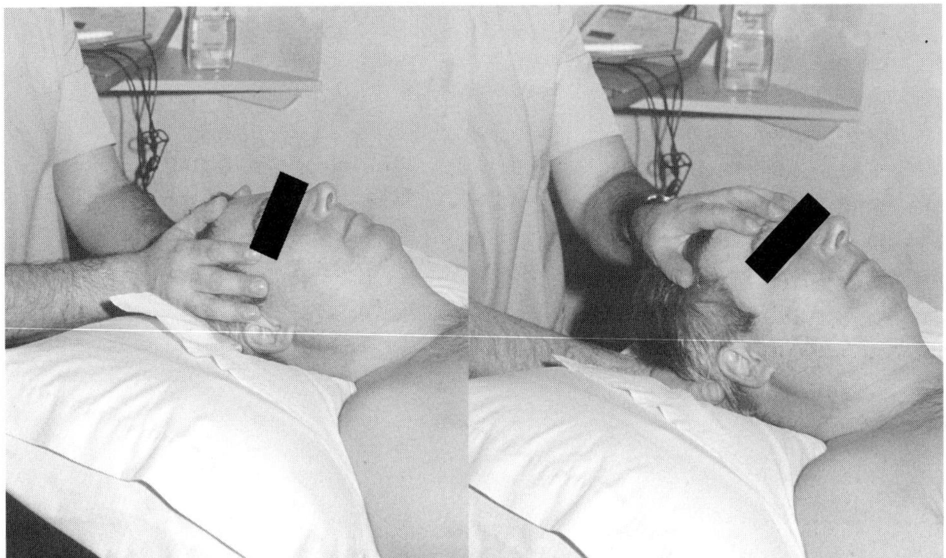

Figure 23. *Cranial treatment.*
The osteopath's hand is placed in two different positions, cradling the head laterally and antero-posteriorly. The cranial procedure involves very gentle pressure and minimal movements.

flexion (inspiration) phase and an extension (expiration) phase, faintly changing the shape of the ventricles. Similar to the thoracic duct pump exerting an influence upon the entire lymphatic system, the CRI can be palpated throughout the body.

The main cranial technique I use is a procedure known as a CV4 (the compression of the fourth ventricle). This compression is achieved by gentle force applied with both hands, pressing medially at the lateral angles of the occiput.

It is my belief that by using the CV4 technique, the volume within the fourth ventricle is reduced, forcing the cerebrospinal fluid out; by this means, drainage through the cribriform plate and down the spine is enhanced. Accordingly, the technique plays an important part in overall treatment.

Care should be taken not to over-stimulate the cranial rhythm with too long or forceful a treatment. After resuming a seated position, the patient is advised to remain sitting for a moment and not to stand abruptly. This is aimed at reducing dizziness due to the neural mediated hypotension commonly found in CFS/ME (see Chapter 5).

This first section of Chapter 10 has touched upon the osteopathic techniques I use in the treatment of CFS/ME. Some of the excellent books written about the entire spectrum of osteopathic techniques are listed in the Further Reading section at the end of the book.

Self-help advice

Osteopathic treatment is not synonymous with manipulation. Many treatments of numerous conditions would be found to be insufficient if they relied on manual therapy alone.[2] As in standard osteopathic practice, advice is given to patients to help improve their general health.

Dorsal rotation exercise

I have observed that manual treatment improves function of the thorax and the spine, especially when enhanced by routine mobility exercises. An effective exercise prescribed to improve and maintain the quality of movement of the dorsal spine is as follows (see Figs 24, 25 and 26):

1. The patient should be seated and place his/her hands around the side of the neck (see Fig 24). S/he should slowly rotate the trunk, together with the head and neck. This gentle rotation is designed not to stretch muscles and joints, but gradually and subtly to increase movement of the upper thoracic vertebrae. The arc of rotation should be only about 45 degrees in total from right to left. This should be repeated five times each way, without stopping in the middle. The movement must be rhythmic, with the patient feeling relaxed throughout the process.
2. The patient should cross his/her arms and hug his/her shoulders with his/her hands (see Fig 25). The movement to the right and left should be repeated five times each way as above, making sure that the head, neck and shoulders all move in unison. This part of the exercise encourages movement in the middle section of the thoracic spine.
3. With the patient remaining seated, the exercise should be repeated, once again five times each way, with the arms folded at the waist (see Fig 26). Rotating the trunk in this position improves mobility of the lower dorsal and upper lumbar segments of the spine.

Patients should carry out the entire sequence three times a day. Since it is a very gentle exercise, even severe CFS/ME should not prevent the patient from doing the exercise. However, the patient is advised to cease exercises if pain develops at any

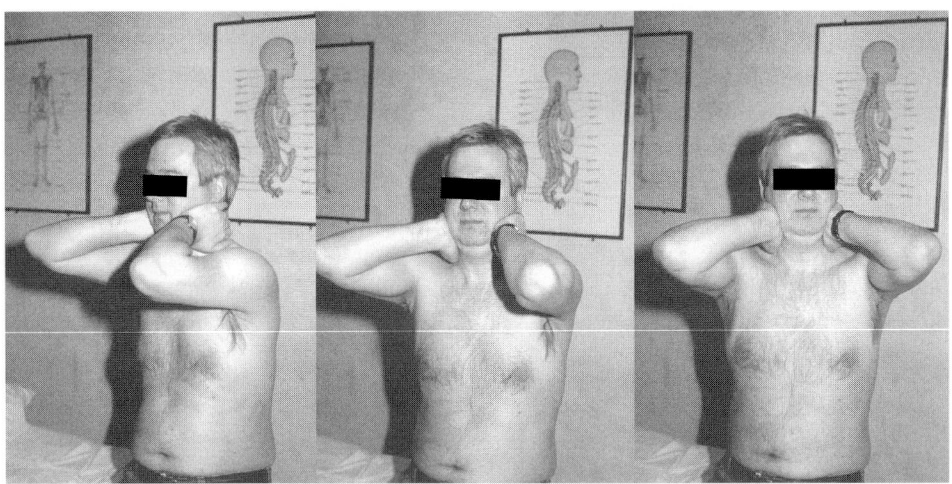

Figure 24. *Upper thoracic rotation exercise.*
The patient slowly rotates his upper back five times each way, through an arc of 45 degrees while sitting. When holding the side of his neck, the patient finds that this rotation gently stretches the upper thoracic spine.

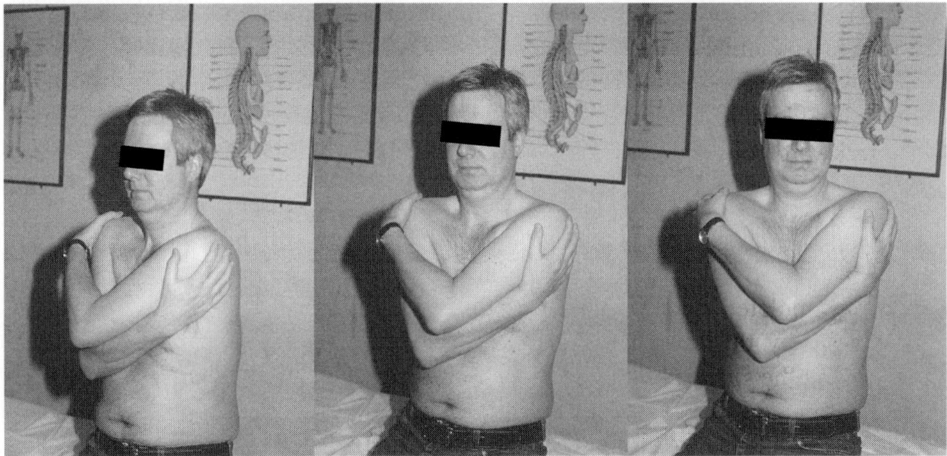

Figure 25. *Mid-thoracic rotation exercise.*
The patient slowly rotates his back five times each way, through an arc of 45 degrees while sitting. When holding the shoulders, this rotation exercise gently stretches the mid-thoracic spine.

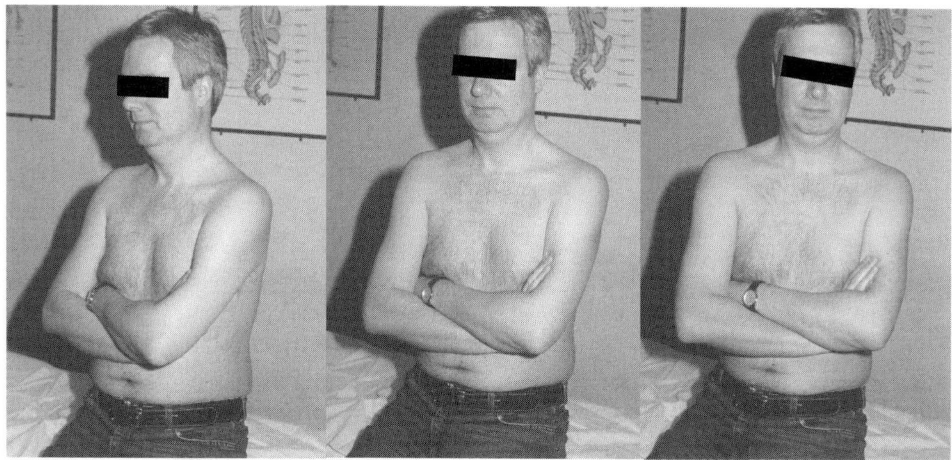

Figure 26. *Lower thoracic rotation exercise.*
The patient slowly rotates his back five times each way, through an arc of 45 degrees while sitting. When folding the arms, the patient finds that this rotation exercise gently stretches the lower thoracic spine.

time during or following the routine. The complete routine in all three positions takes about one minute, when performed at the correct speed.

Following the above exercise, the patient is advised to stand up, and gently shrug his/her shoulders, rolling them slowly forward five times and then slowly repeating with backward rolls five times. This exercise should be carried out at least three times a day (see Fig. 27).

Cross-crawl

One can stimulate both halves of the brain to work together in harmony with the whole body by the exercise known as cross-crawl. The cross-crawl exercise is marching on the spot. The marching action should be slow and deliberate, with the patient's right arm moving in unison with the left leg. This action is repeated, moving the left arm forward together with the right leg. CFS/ME patients usually find this simple task difficult to perform at the beginning of therapy, since their bodies are so un-coordinated. It is very important not to move the arm and leg of the same side together, as this will succeed in throwing the body (and mind) further out of balance. After practising for a while, patients are able to carry out the cross-crawl

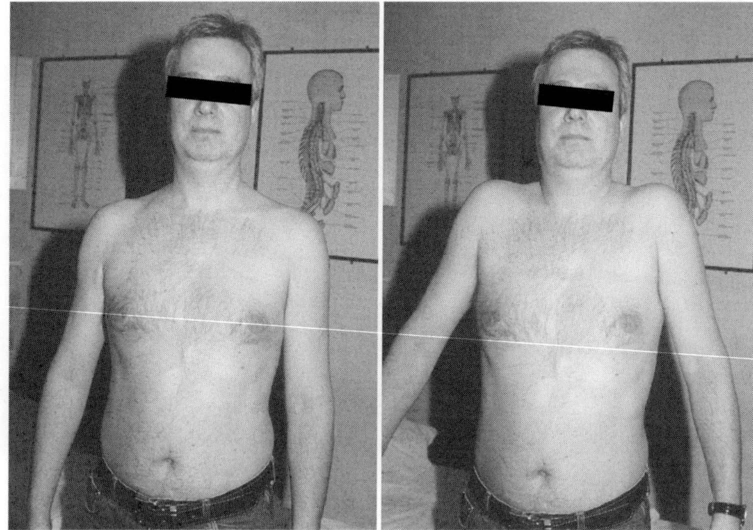

Figure 27. *Shoulder shrug exercise.*
While standing, the patient gently shrugs his shoulders, rolling them slowly forward five times and then slowly repeating with backward rolls five times.

exercise without much difficulty. The marching routine is to be done for up to five minutes in total in an entire day, a minute or so at a time. Any exercises that overexert the patient are to be avoided.

Self-massage routine

The patient is advised to aid the lymphatic drainage of the head and spine through a self-massage routine.

Nasal release

This massage schedule begins with the patient, seated, applying gentle pressure to open the junction between the forehead and nose and aid drainage into the mucous membrane of the nasal sinuses. The minimal force required is accomplished by mildly pressing the pads of both second fingers up against the inner canthus (inside corner of the eye) or conversely, pulling slightly down just above the bridge of the nose. The patient should choose the technique with which s/he feels most comfortable and which enables him/her to breathe easily through the nose. During the first ten days of self-treatment, the pressure with the fingers should be held for a seven-minute period. This has been shown to bring about a lasting release of the region by enhancing breathing and lymphatic drainage. After the first ten days, patients should continue with nasal release for a one-minute period each day in order to maintain the improvement (see Fig. 28).

Facial massage

The patient, while remaining seated, should gently stroke the fingertips of one spread hand down his/her faces to the chin (see Fig. 29). This gentle facial effleurage should be carried out for twenty seconds with a rate of one stroke roughly every four seconds.

Head massage

The above gentle stroking method should be repeated for twenty seconds at a time on both sides and the back of the head down to the neck (see Fig. 30).

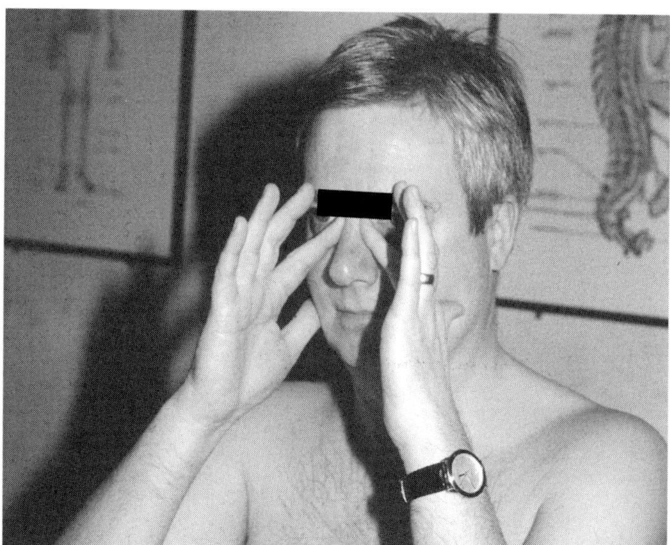

Figure 28. *Nasal release.*
The seated patient gently presses the pads of both second digits up against the inner canthus (inside corner of the eye) or conversely, pulls slightly down just above the bridge of the nose.

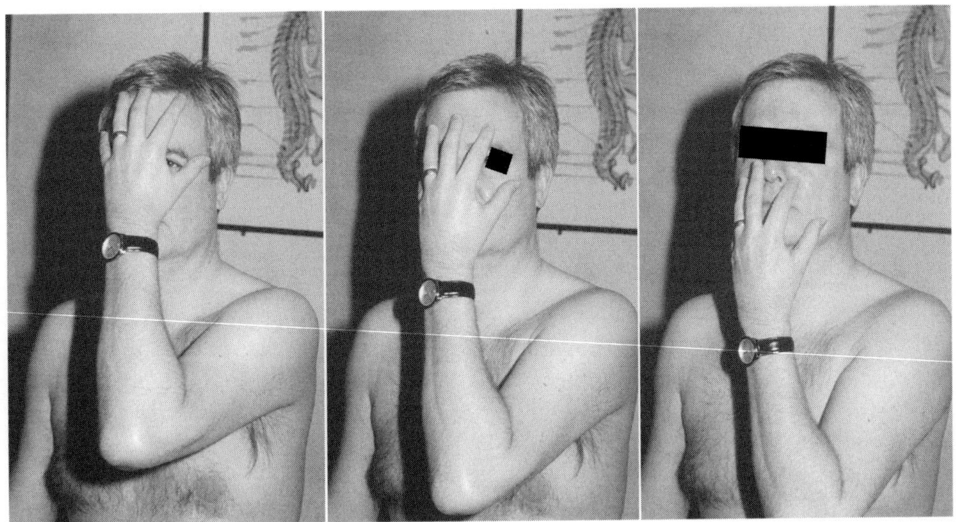

Figure 29. *Facial self massage.*
The patient gently strokes the fingertips of one spread hand down his face to the chin for twenty seconds.

Anterior neck massage

The patient should lie down and, using almond oil or baby oil, continue with bilateral effleurage of the neck down to the clavicles (shoulder blades) for twenty seconds each side (see Fig. 31)

Breast massage

The patient massages the lateral, central and medial sections of the breast in turn for twenty seconds, with a slow rhythmic stroking manoeuvre up towards the clavicles, thus directing the lymph away from the axillary (in the arm pits) lymph nodes to avoid risk of glandular swelling (see Fig. 32).

Back massage

Having adopted a prone position, the patient receives back massage from a family member or friend. The massage routine consists of one minute of gentle upward effleurage to the sides of the spine, finishing in the shoulder region at a level with

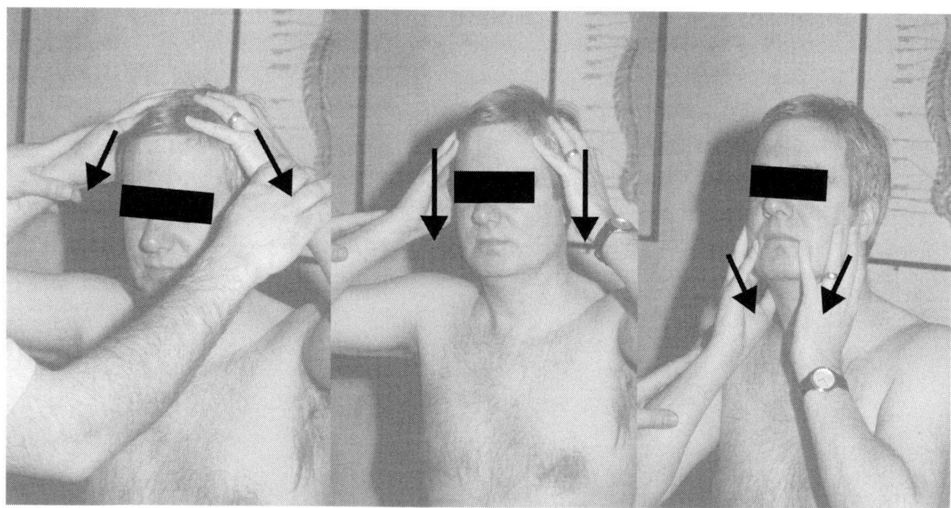

Figure 30. *Self massage to head.*
The patient gently strokes the fingers of both spread hands down the sides of his head to the neck for twenty seconds.

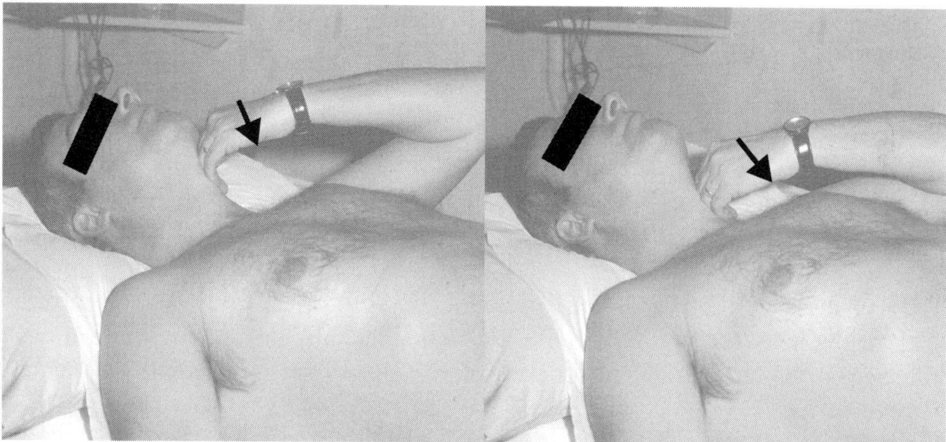

Figure 31. *Anterior neck self massage.*
The arrows show the direction of the self-massage technique, which is always towards each clavicle, on both sides for twenty seconds. The pressure applied by the patient should be much less than during a treatment session, concentrating only on the superficial lymphatics in the self-massage.

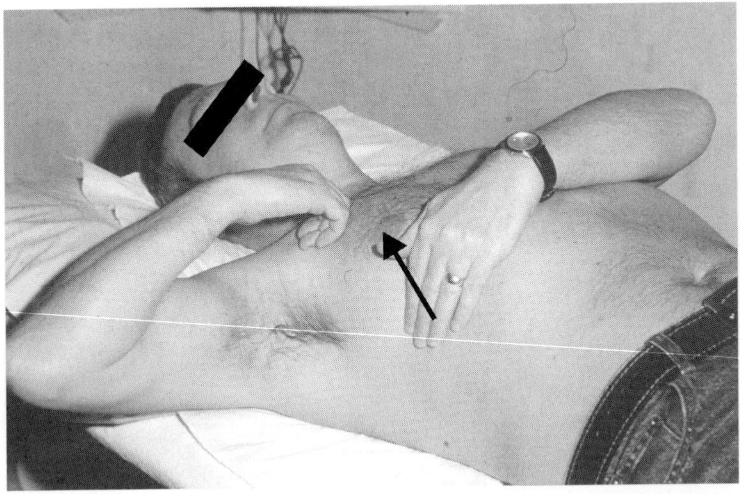

Figure 32. *Self massage of the breast.*
The arrows show the direction of the self-massage technique. The patient massages the lateral, central and medial sections of each breast in turn for twenty seconds, with a slow rhythmic stroking manoeuvre up towards the clavicles. The pressure applied by the patient should be much less than during a treatment session, concentrating only on the superficial lymphatics in the self massage.

the clavicles. If no help is available from another individual, patients should use back brushes to accomplish the back massage.

Posterior neck massage

The self-massage routine should be completed with downward effleurage of the back of the neck for twenty seconds on both sides, just in case the upward back massage is too vigorous and upward pressure is applied too high above the clavicles.

Returning to good health

Patients are advised to avoid any stress whether physical, mental or emotional whenever possible. Activities that exert strain on the body are to be avoided. If the patient's occupation involves too much physical activity, they are advised to stop work temporarily or reduce their workload. This especially applies to tasks that put extra mechanical strain on the thoracic spine.

Physical tasks that exert too much strain on the patient are, if possible, to be done by a helpful colleague. Members of the patient's family are advised to share the workload at home, to make life as bearable as possible, until treatment has restored the sufferer to better health.

If the patient usually spends time in front of a computer or if they are desk-bound at work, they are advised to stand up every half-hour for a minute or two, and walk around the office. They should also take a fifteen-minute break every two hours.

The patient is instructed to avoid slumping into a soft chair. When relaxing, patients are advised to lie on their side on a couch or a bed with their head well supported and a pillow between their knees. Lying on the side puts minimal strain on the spine.

Patients are advised to vary their diet as much as possible. This reduces the possibility of placing strain on any particular region of the gastrointestinal system. Processed foods are to be avoided and wholemeal flour and brown sugar should replace the white variety. Stimulants such as caffeine are to be avoided particularly in CFS/ME. Decaffeinated coffee and decaffeinated tea or herbal tea can be drunk instead, but, because decaffeinated coffee has been shown to increase cholesterol levels, this should be taken only in moderation.

Patients should eat regular, healthy meals and drink plenty of healthy fluids, preferably mineral or filtered water – 2 litres a day should be enough. The intake of tobacco, alcohol and too much medication may exert a strain on the gut, and thus the sympathetic nervous system. This will undoubtedly make the symptoms of CFS/ME worse. Smoking, drinking alcohol and the taking of medication should be kept to a minimum, and avoided completely if possible.

As well as a healthy diet, I prescribe a supplement of vitamins C and B complex. The former increases the patient's resistance to infection, while B complex improves general functioning of the nervous system. A high dose vitamin C pill of 1000 mg is recommended three times a week and a strong, or whole B complex tablet once a day. Vitamins B and C are both water-soluble so that any excess is excreted from the body and cannot be stored. However, as there is a risk of developing kidney stones if the vitamin C intake is too high or if the patient suffers from kidney disease, it is wise not to take the 1000 mg pill every day.

Beware of taking so many different supplements that any possible benefit is likely to be outweighed by undesirable side-effects (see Fig. 33), EPA and virgin evening primrose oil excepted.

Even though excessive supplements are harmful, occasionally they may be needed. If a patient develops a cold or flu, it is a sign that the immune system is starting to work properly. In the early stages of CFS/ME there is an upward regulation of the immune response, so, while a patient with CFS/ME rarely experiences colds or flu, they just feel constantly ill. Eventually, as the system balances, there is more and more chance of developing colds and other upper respiratory tract infections.

For colds and flu

I recommend a combination of Echinacea – a good natural immune system stimulant, one of nature's natural antibiotics – bee propolis, and the most effective

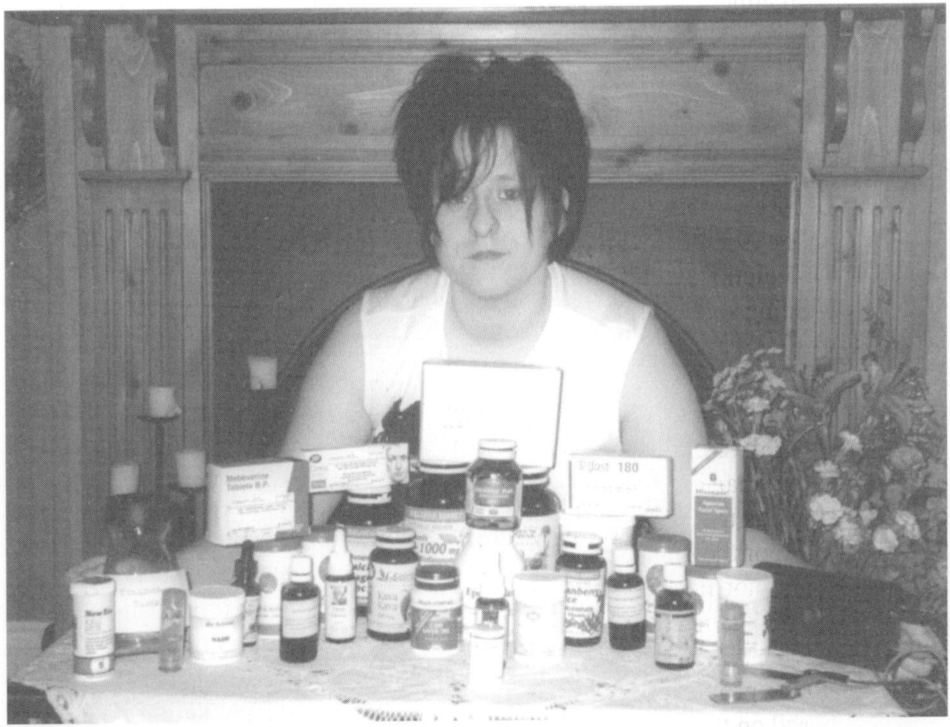

Figure 33. *A CFS/ME patient and her daily medication.*

and probably the most hideous tasting antioxidant, grapefruit seed extract, known as citracidal.

Flu jabs are at the patient's discretion. Some vaccines, including the flu vaccine, contain mercury so you should be wary, but some patients' immune systems are very poor. These tend to be the very severe long-term sufferers who struggle to respond to treatment. Immunisation in these cases may be the only option.

Sleep can sometimes be helped by having an extra small meal an hour before going to bed. As the hypothalamus controls sleep as well as satiety and hunger, this sometimes tricks it into switching on the sleep centres. Self-hypnosis also can often help the patient switch off and relieve sleep problems.

Frequency of treatment

At the beginning of treatment it is important that the patient is treated once a week and that the treatment remains regular and weekly. This usually continues for the first 12 weeks and, slowly, as symptoms improve, there is a gradual increase in the time between consultations. With very severe cases, weekly treatments may be necessary for much longer than three months. Eventually, when patients remain symptom-free between their six monthly check-ups and are able to perform all reasonable activities with no after-effects, I will score them 10 out of 10 and they are pronounced cured. While acknowledging that every patient is different, I have devised a chart (see Table 2, page 114) that is a guide to both the patient and practitioner predicting the likely length of treatment.

This is a sliding scale and should be used as a general guide only, as there may be other factors to take into account. In other words, if at the start of treatment a patient is scored 5/10 on CFS/ME, but is also suffering from another disorder, the overall score may be 4/10 or lower. If the physical findings during the examination are very pronounced, the overall score is lowered. I often find that the patient is trying to appear healthier than s/he really is. This fits the profile of most CFS/ME sufferers who try as hard as they can to keep going until, eventually, they have to admit they cannot carry on or they just collapse.

The body cannot lie and, after physically examining the patient together with taking a detailed history, the trained practitioner should be able to give a reasonably accurate score that informs the patient how long the treatment programme may take. As the treatment progresses and the symptoms improve, a periodic reassessment of the score, based on the symptoms and physical signs, is useful.

It is a wonderful feeling for both sufferer and practitioner when a patient's score is 10/10. This means that, without any treatment in the previous six months, the patient is and has been totally symptom-free, and, in addition, has been able to do everything s/he could do before s/he was ill, within reason, without suffering any side effects. The patient is then discharged.

Annual check-up

Whether the treatment proves to be a lasting cure or just remission depends on many factors that will affect the patient after being discharged. If the patient habitually overstrains their body, s/he may experience the return of symptoms. The patient should seek treatment as soon as the symptoms reappear in order to avoid a long-lasting relapse. The predisposition to developing CFS/ME takes the form of a disturbed

Table 2 The outlook

Score	Description	Prognosis
1	Extreme symptoms and signs for more than a year. Totally bed-ridden or sitting all day, little cranial flow palpable.	3 years +
2	Severe symptoms and signs for more than a year. Bed-ridden or sitting all day, little cranial flow palpable.	2 years+
3	Severe symptoms and signs for more than a year, resting most of the day, little cranial flow palpable.	2 years
4	Severe symptoms and signs for 6–12 months, resting most of the day, little cranial flow palpable.	18 months+
5	Severe symptoms and signs for at least 6 months; able to carry out light tasks but requires regular rest periods.	12–18 months
6	Moderate symptoms and signs for at least 6 months; able to work part-time with a struggle.	8–12 months
7	Moderate symptoms and signs for at least 6 months; able to work full time with difficulty.	8 months
8	Moderate symptoms and signs for at least 6 months; daily life slightly limited. Symptoms worsen on activity.	6 months
9	No symptoms but still signs of slight lymphatic engorgement and experiences mild symptoms following over-exertion	3 months
10	Symptom-free for at least 6 months. Able to live a full active life …within reason.	Discharged

drainage system and consequently, the patient should continue the dorsal rotation exercises for life after being discharged, and occasionally, maybe once a week, do the self-massage routine in the shower. Annual check-ups are a good idea, although I appreciate that some patients prefer to put the whole episode behind them.

Toxins in the brain don't cause pain

One indication that the Perrin Technique is not a placebo is the fact that most patients feel a great deal worse at the beginning of their treatment. Placebo treatments do not, generally, make you feel worse. The reason for this initial exacerbation in the symptoms is due to the fact that, for the first time, the toxins embedded (possibly for years) in the central nervous system are being released into the rest of the body.

The most common symptoms in the early stages are nausea, headaches and general pain. These complaints can be easily explained. Nausea is caused, usually, by the liver having to cope with the extra toxins, which are draining via the lymphatic drainage into the blood. This is why I advise patients to take milk thistle extract (silymarin) and plenty of drinking water, as they are useful in helping the liver cope with the increased level of toxins. If you cannot tolerate milk thistle, try ginger. Those patients who cannot cope with any supplements should drink plenty of water and follow as healthy and balanced a diet as possible.

If patients have a dental appointment, they should remember the instructions given in Chapter 7 (see page 66), regarding type of filling and anaesthetic.

Headaches and pain may also be due to excess toxicity. As the treatment encourages the toxins to leave the brain, the toxins will initially affect the superficial tissues in the head and, as they drain down to the rest of the body, pain may follow. The toxins inside the brain do not cause pain as there are no pain receptors within the brain. However, toxins *do* affect the function of the brain, and this accounts for most of the symptoms of CFS/ME.

The first few weeks, or sometimes months in severe cases, are always the most trying for the patients. The worse the patient is in the early stages of treatment, the better, usually, it bodes for their prognosis.

While the body's drainage system is improving with the treatment, another unpleasant sign is the appearance of spots, boils and other skin eruptions. Until the lymphatic channels are working properly, the toxins have to go somewhere and the quickest way out of the body is often through the skin. These skin problems normally clear up as the treatment progresses.

The main aspects for CFS/ME sufferers to focus upon are the changes occurring with the treatment. (If change has not occurred in any way during the first twelve weeks of treatment, the patient may have to take an alternative route in their search for a cure.) My treatment often hugely improves the patient's health, but some may need other treatments in tandem in order to alleviate all symptoms. I have noticed that other treatments – whether they are dietetically or pharmacologically based – work better after the patient's neurolymphatic pathways have been improved. Patients who have tried supplements before treatment to no avail, are advised to try some of the supplements again after undergoing the Perrin Technique, as they may now prove more effective.

Remember that there are other conditions that can commonly occur together with CFS/ME that may require an additional or slightly different approach. For example, fibromyalgia is often seen in CFS/ME patients. This condition, which features painful muscles, can be detected by palpating 18 known trigger points throughout the body. If at least 11 of the 18 are tender, fibromyalgia is diagnosed. There are many books on the subject with illustrations of the trigger points. Because the massage used in my treatment plan may aggravate the pain in fibromyalgia, the massage should be kept to the minimum in these cases. The painful joints should be gently stretched with plenty of cold compresses laid only on the spine (cold, not frozen, ice pops placed longitudinally are useful for this) and warm compresses placed on the surrounding paravertebral muscles.

CFS/ME in children

There are thousands of childhood cases of CFS/ME a year recorded in the UK. However, you rarely see children younger than five with the condition,[5] due to the fact that CFS/ME (1) takes time to develop and (2) is linked to postural problems in the spine, affecting the body's drainage of toxins. A child starts to walk at about one year and it takes a few years to develop a painful, bad posture. A major spinal trauma may precipitate the onset of CFS/ME in the very young, but this is extremely rare.

It is difficult to persuade children to reduce their level of activity when they want to do so much. It is hard to help the parents maintain a positive attitude when, initially, they may see their child becoming more ill. However, some patients do improve immediately, for patients do not necessarily get worse before starting to recover. One patient improved so quickly that within weeks he was able to take up football and tennis; I think it was lucky that I treated him at just the right time for the body quickly and safely to return to normal. However, most patients are not that fortunate and may suffer to begin with during treatment. Often the parent looks at me, thinking, perhaps, 'What are you doing to my child?'

I have a great deal of sympathy with the parents of any sick child. CFS/ME affects the whole family, so I often try to have as many members of the family as possible at the consultation so that they can understand what is going on.

Our son, Max

I empathise with parents who see their lovely child go from a healthy, active boy or girl to a wheelchair-bound invalid. When my son, Max, was only five, he started exhibiting signs and symptoms of fatigue. My wife and I began to be concerned when he complained of constant headaches. We became very worried when he started projectile vomiting every morning and so we took him to our GP who referred him to the hospital. There he was examined by a paediatrician and a trainee doctor who refused to scan his brain, saying that it was a virus. I told them that I had spent years studying the brain and that his signs bore the hallmarks of increased intracranial pressure. He had banged his head a week before and I was concerned that this was the reason. They took a chest X-ray, but refused a scan and sent us home. Another two trips to the doctor's and we were again told that it was a virus. One doctor said remarkably to me that Max, who by then had to be carried into the surgery, was suffering from 'sibling rivalry': his little brother was born the year that Max fell ill, so, maintained the doctor, he was seeking attention.

A week later he was undergoing surgery to remove a pylocytic astrocytoma from his cerebellum or, to put it into lay terms, a tumour from the back of his brain. The pressure caused by the tumour had damaged the ventricular system in the brain, affecting the drainage of cerebrospinal fluid. He therefore required a further operation in which the surgeons implanted a ventricular peritoneal shunt. This is a tube with a valve, placed under the skin, which drains the cerebrospinal fluid from the brain to the abdomen where it is absorbed back into the blood.

Watching a child suffer – even when the techniques and operations are life-saving – is an experience that no parent should have to endure. I fully understand the anxieties of young patients' parents and the long wait for the child to start to recover. Seeing the child re-emerge from CFS/ME is an exhilarating experience, both for parents and the practitioner, and helps maintain the practitioner's enthusiasm during the long and sometimes arduous treatment programme.

It *will* get better

As I have already said, while a patient is on the road to recovery, certain additional signs and symptoms may be seen and pain experienced. This is usually a case of it gets worse before it gets better.

Despite these unpleasant signs and symptoms initially, it is now only a matter of time for most CFS/ME sufferers before my treatment starts to work and the characteristics of this debilitating disease begin to recede.

Chapter 11

Recovery and prevention

Science is nothing but trained and organised common sense.
Thomas Henry Huxley (1825–1895)

CFS/ME can affect all ages and all cultures, men as well as women, but many more women suffer from the disease than men. This is because (1) women's hormonal systems are so much more complex than men's and those hormonal changes affect CFS/ME[1] and (2) there is much more lymphatic tissue in the breast in women and thus there is much more congestion of the tissue in the chest, irritating more of the sympathetic nerves in this important area.[2]

Causes

There are many factors involved in the process leading to CFS/ME, as discussed in earlier chapters. The head may be traumatised at birth or there may be a genetic predisposition that affects the normal development of the head or back.[3] Years before the onset of symptoms, perhaps even in early childhood, the patient may have suffered from trauma to the head or spine. Teenage years bring with them problems of their own and the spine of a very active teenager, or of those who tend to slouch when sitting, is prone to developmental problems.

One of the functions of the cerebrospinal fluid is drainage. Some poisons caused by infection, inflammation or toxins from the polluted environment enter the brain and spine and flow out through perforations in the skull and minute channels in the spine, entering the lymphatic system.[4] If there are structural problems affecting both the head and the spine together, there is no safe drainage pathway for the cerebrospinal fluid to take. In a CFS/ME sufferer these normal drainage points are congested, leading to a build-up of poisons within the central nervous system.[2]

The main organ in the brain to be affected by poisons is the hypothalamus, which is the control centre for the hormones and the sympathetic nervous system. The latter helps the body cope in times of stress. In CFS/ME the toxic cocktail brewing in the hypothalamus leads to an overload of the sympathetic nervous system, which will have been affected by other stress factors – whether physical, allergic, emotional or infection – in the years leading up to the illness.[5,6]

One final trigger, which is usually a viral or bacterial infection, will lead to a breakdown in the normal functioning of the sympathetic nervous system.[5] Furthermore, the lymphatic system, which is meant to aid drainage, is controlled by the sympathetic nervous system.[7] When this system is functioning poorly, toxins are pumped in the reverse direction, which adds further poisons to the central nervous system. As the toxicity builds up, brain function worsens, leading to further sympathetic disarray. The vicious circle that ensues leads to the myriad symptoms affecting the patient with CFS/ME.[2]

Treatment

The Perrin Technique stimulates the motion of fluid around the brain and spinal cord via cranial techniques[8] (see Chapter 10). Treatment to the spine, as well as certain exercises, further aids drainage of these toxins out of the cerebrospinal fluid.[9] Massage of the soft tissues in the head, neck, back and chest directs all the poisons out of the lymphatic system and into the blood, and eventually to the liver where they are broken down and readily detoxified.[10]

Eventually, with no poisons affecting the central nervous system, the hypothalamus and the sympathetic nerves start to work better, gradually stimulating improved lymphatic drainage. Thus the body starts to function correctly and, providing patients do not overstrain themselves as the nervous system is recovering, their symptoms should gradually improve.

'The rule of the artery reigns supreme.' This tenet was formulated by the founder of osteopathy, Dr Andrew Taylor Still, who stated that illness is mainly due to stagnation of body fluids and that if you can stimulate blood flow and other fluid motion, including cerebrospinal fluid and lymphatic drainage, the body will recover.[10]

My method of treating CFS/ME, using the principle above, is analogous to mending a blocked main drain in your home. By increasing pressure into the main drain, one pumps out the blockage. It is obviously more complex in the body and the techniques do not actually unblock the thoracic duct, the body's main drain, but by cranial treatment, articulation of the spine and manual lymphatic drainage massage, one stimulates the movement of cerebrospinal fluid from the brain and the spine to the lymphatics. This increases pressure and thus improves the movement of lymph fluid from the thoracic duct into the bloodstream, from where it will eventually detoxify in the liver.[2]

Responses to treatment

The most common symptoms in the early stages of treatment include nausea, headaches, general pain and the appearance of spots and boils.[2] (See pages 115–116.) My experience has shown that the worse the patient becomes in the early stage of treatment, the better the overall prognosis is likely to be. What matters is the change that occurs with the treatment. If change has not occurred in any way in the first twelve weeks, it does not mean that the patient has no hope of recovery but it may mean they have to seek an alternative therapy in their search for a cure. Some fortunate patients do improve immediately, so it is not necessarily the case that a CFS/ME patient's condition worsens before improving.[11]

Treatment schedule

At the beginning of treatment, the patient is treated once a week. As the symptom picture improves, there should be a gradual increase in the period between consultations.

Week 1–12	weekly
Week 13–24	every 2 weeks
Week 25–36	every 3 weeks
Week 36–52	every 4 weeks
Month 12–18	every 3 months
Month 24	final check-up (if symptom-free for 6 months, patient is discharged).

The recovery process

Once patients have noticed a reduction in their symptoms, they can begin the uphill battle to improve their health and stamina. They have first to convalesce. Convalescence is no longer a fashionable concept. People having some operations nowadays tend to be discharged from hospital within a day and may be at work within the week. Convalescent rest, however, is a must during the process of recovery from CFS/ME.

In order to turn the remission period in CFS/ME into a permanent cure, as well as convalescence patients must keep to the half rule until they are symptom-free for at least six months. As I tell my patients, 'remember that half of more is still more!' In other words, as you recover and can do more before fatigue sets in, you should only gradually increase activity, while still taking care to avoid too much exertion. Double the effort may prove possible but at this stage it is not advisable.

Climbing the recovery mountain carries its own hazards. When one is very poorly with any protracted illness, the recovery mountain exists, but one is too ill to notice or care, so one passes it by; it has no relevance to the day-to-day existence of the sufferer. When one embarks on a treatment programme and symptoms start to improve, it is akin to climbing that mountain. As patients get higher and higher, they look down and feel sad and depressed that they were so ill. When they look up, their anxiety increases as they realise how much further they have to go until they reach the summit. So, patients' moods will often change as they improve. It was noticeable, in the clinical trials, that as the treated patients' fatigue, pain and cognitive function improved, in the early stages their anxiety and depression scores worsened.[11] This, at least, showed that CFS/ME is not a psychological disorder in which the other symptoms correspond to depression or anxiety scores.

With treatment and exercise, the patient will gradually improve and, as time goes by, will become capable of leading a more active life. Patients who are eager to resume sports should begin by gentle walks up and down the road and gradually build up the distance.

Swimming is of benefit when the patient feels ready, preferably gentle backstroke. Breast stroke should be avoided as it exerts too much pressure on the spine with the stretch of the neck and the kicking of the legs. I recommend backstroke with low rhythmic up and down movements of the legs and with sidestrokes of the arms, as in sculling. This will improve joint mobility and increase the tone of the muscles throughout the body.

As the symptoms continue to improve, both the patient and the practitioner will be greatly encouraged. By steadily improving the mobility of the spine, and by relaxing all the irritated surrounding tissues, the function of the sympathetic nervous system should finally be restored to full working order. The patient once again enjoys health, vigour and a good quality of life.

Avoid toxins

All of us are exposed to many pollutants in our everyday lives. CFS/ME sufferers need to minimise as far as possible their exposure to these toxins. (See Chapter 7 for a detailed list.)

Avoid having further mercury amalgam dental fillings.[12] When visiting the hair salon, the use of chemicals in your hair should be limited.[13] Remember that the scalp is very close to the brain and it is not advisable to massage poisons into the skin in this area. Take care to make sure that your neck is in a comfortable position, too, when your hair is being washed in a back basin.

If you live in the countryside, take a trip away from home during crop spraying days.[14] If your work entails working with harmful toxins, you may want to consider a career change.

Recurrence

As patients recover, if they overdo things, suffer from infections or have to cope with too much stress, their symptoms may return or get worse. Some patients do suffer recurrences when they have significantly improved, but few experience relapse once they have been discharged, unless they push themselves too far day after day. CFS/ME patients, once recovered, need to reassess their lifestyle and take steps to reduce the continual stress that may have partly led to the illness in the first place. They should be able to exert themselves when cured, but knowing when to stop is important.

Patients who are discharged should continue the dorsal rotation exercises three times a day for life. Self-massage to the chest and neck should be done once a week in the shower. An annual check-up is advisable.

Should a relapse occur, it might take a long time to reverse, but remember, if the treatment worked the first time, it can work again and perhaps more quickly the second time. Psychologists and counsellors are invaluable in these cases. The important rule in treatment, and even more so after relapse, is to remain as positive as possible. To secure a permanent remission and to remain in good health, you have to focus on the task ahead by means of sensible pacing. Once better, follow a graded exercise programme thus achieving a slow, sure return to good health.

Prevention

I am one of the few practitioners who maintain that CFS/ME can be prevented. The physical signs are very real and usually are seen long before the symptoms begin (see Chapter 8). This is why in the very early stages of the disorder only a physical and postural-based examination can detect the development of this disorder before the sympathetic nervous system breaks down.

If CFS/ME is found in more than one family member, there may be a genetic predisposition that leads to a restricted flow of toxins from the brain and spine. I have observed this genetic factor many times where the children or siblings of the patient show very early signs of fatigue. Sometimes the family member may suffer only from chronic infections but nothing more specific, and yet, on examination, they have all the physical signs of CFS/ME, which quickly disappear with only a few weeks or months of treatment. For these reasons, I believe that CFS/ME is preventable if treated and managed properly in the early stages.

Most leading authorities agree that the quicker that CFS/ME is diagnosed and treatment starts, together with avoiding overstrain on the body, the better the chances of recovery are. The very severe cases of patients in bed 24/7 in silent, darkened rooms should never happen. This may occur as a result of inappropriate treatment being given in the early stages of the illness, with patients being advised and sometimes coerced to increase their activity, and/or being wrongly medicated. I believe early rest, pacing at the outset, together with prompt treatment to restore a healthy lymphatic and nervous system, will one day make CFS/ME an illness of the past.

Further Reading

Appenzeller O. *The Autonomic Nervous System. An introduction to basic and clinical concepts*. 4th edition. New York, Elsevier; 1990.

Bannister Sir R, and Mathias C, (Eds.). *Autonomic Failure*. 3rd edition. Oxford: Oxford Medical; 1993.

Browse N, Burnand KG, Mortimer PS. *Diseases of the Lymphatics*. London: Hodder Arnold; 2003.

Chaitow L. *Fibromyalgia Syndrome. A Practitioner's Guide to Treatment*. Edinburgh, Churchill Livingstone; 2000.

Chaitow L. *Cranial manipulation: Theory and practice*. New York, Elsevier; 2005.

Chickly B. *Silent Waves, Theory and Practice of Lymph Drainage Therapy.* 2nd edition. Scottsdale, AZ: I.H.H Publishing; 2004.

Ellenhorn MJ, (Ed.). *Ellenhorn's Medical Toxicology: Diagnosis and Treatment of Human Poisoning*. 2nd edition. Philadelphia; Williams & Wilkins; 1997.

Gershon MD. *The Second Brain. New York: Harper Perennial; 1999.*

Goldstein J. *Chronic Fatigue Syndromes: The Limbic Hypothesis.* New York: The Haworth Medical Press; 1993.

Hartman L. Handbook of Osteopathic Technique (3rd revised edition). London: Nelson Thornes; 1996.

Kinmonth JB. *The Lymphatics*. 2nd edition. London: Edward Arnold; 1982.

Lay EM. *Cranial Field: Foundations for Osteopathic Medicine*. Philadelpia: Williams and Wilkins; 1997.

Lewis T. *The Soldier's Heart and the Effort Syndrome*. New York: Paul B. Hober; 1920.

Loeser JD, Butler SH, Chapman RC, Turk DC (Eds.) *Bonica's Management of Pain*. 3rd edition. Philadelphia: Lippincott, Williams & Wilkins; 2001.

Macintyre A. *ME, Post-viral Fatigue Syndrome: How to Live with it*. 2nd edition. Thorsons; 1992.

McKone WL. *Osteopathic medicine: philosophy, principles, and practice*. Oxford: Blackwell Science; 2001.

Miller JB. Intradermal provocative-neutralizing food testing and subcutaneous food extract injection therapy. In: Brostoff J & Challacombe SJ (Eds.) *Food Allergy and Intolerance* London: Baillière Tindall; 1987.

Nathan B. *Touch and Emotion in Manual Therapy*. Edinburgh: Churchill Livingstone; 1999. Pellegrino MJ. *Post-traumatic fibromyalgia a medical perspective*. Columbus, OH: Anadem Publishing; 1996.

Pellegrino MJ. *Fibromyalgia: Up Close & Personal*. Columbus, OH: Anadem Pub; 2005.

Pentreath VW (Ed.) *Neurotoxicology in Vitro*. London: CRC Press; 1999.

Puri BK. *Chronic Fatigue Syndrome, a natural way to treat M.E.* London: Hammersmith Press; 2005.

Rea W. *Chemical sensitivity*. Boca Raton, Florida: Lewis Pub; 1993.

Richards J. *Functional Biomechanics in Clinic and Research*. www.biomechanics.org.uk; 1999.

Rogers S. *Tired or Toxic*. New York: Prestige Publishing; 1990.

Sammut E, Searle-Barnes P. *Osteopathic Diagnosis*. Cheltenham: Nelson Thornes; 2002.

Sandler S. *Osteopathy*. (2nd revised edition). London: Vermilion; 1996.

Shepherd C. *Living with M.E., the Chronic Post-viral Syndrome*. London: Vermilion Press; 1998.

Snell RS. *Anatomy for Medical Students*. 5th edition. Philadelphia: Lippincott, Williams and Wilkins; 1995.

Standring S. (Ed.) *Gray's Anatomy,* 39th edition. Edinburgh: Churchill Livingstone; 2004.

Still AT. *Philosophy of Osteopathy*. Published by the Author, Kirksville, Mo; 1899.

Still AT. *The Philosophy and Mechanical Principles of Osteopathy*. Kansas City, MO: Hudson-Kimberly; 1902.

Stoddard A. *Manual of Osteopathic Technique*. 3rd edition. London: Hutchinson; 1982.

Stone C. *Science in the Art of Osteopathy (illustrated)*. Cheltenham: Nelson Thornes; 2000.

Straus S. (Ed.) *Chronic Fatigue Syndrome*. New York: Mark Dekker; 1994.

Sutherland WG. In: Wales AL (Ed.) *Teachings in the Science of Osteopathy*. Ft Worth, Texas: Sutherland Cranial Teaching Foundation; 1990.

Tilson HA, Mitchell CL. *Neurotoxicology*. New York: Raven Press; 1992.

Upledger JE, Vredevoogd JD. *Cranio-Sacral Therapy*. Chicago: Eastland Press; 1983.

Webster GV. *Sage Sayings of Still*. London: Wetzel Publishing Co; 1928.

References

Chapter 1

1. Scwalbe G. *Die Arachnoidairaum ein Lymphraum und sein Zusammenhang mit den Perichorioidairaum.* Zbl med Wiss Zentralblatt fur die medizinschen Wissenschaften. 1869; 7:465–467.
2. Kida S, Pantazis A, Weller RO. CSF Drains Directly from the Subarachnoid space into Nasal Lymphatics in the Rat. Anatomy, Histology and Immunological Significance. *Neuropathology and Applied Neurobiology* 1993; 19: 480–488.
3. Johnston M, Zakharov A, Papaiconomou C, Salmasi G, Armstrong D: Evidence of connections between cerebrospinal fluid and nasal lymphatic vessels in humans, non-human primates and other mammalian species. *Cerebrospinal Fluid Research* 2004; 1: 2.
4. Miura M, Kato S, Von Ludinghausen M. Lymphatic drainage of the cerebrospinal fluid from monkey spinal meninges with special reference to the distribution of epidural lymphatics. *Arch Histol Cytol* 1998; 61: 277–286.
5. Bozanovic Sosic R, Mollanji R, Johnston MG. Spinal and cranial contributions to total cerebrospinal fluid transport. *American Journal of Physiology* 2001; 281, 3–2: R909–R916.
6. Boulton M, Flessner M, Armstrong D, Hay J, Johnston M. Determination of volumetric cerebrospinal fluid absorption into extracranial lymphatics in sheep. *American Journal of Physiology* 1998; 274: 1 (2). R88–96.
7. Bradbury MWB, Cole DF. The role of the lymphatic system in drainage of cerebrospinal fluid and aqueous humour. *Journal of Physiology* 1980; 299: 353–365.

8. Mokri B, Aksamit AJ, Atkinson JL. Paradoxical postural headaches in cerebrospinal fluid leaks. *Cephalalgia* 2004; 24(10):883–7.
9. Czerniaswska A. Experimental investigations on the penetration of 198Au from nasal mucous membrane in to cerebrospinal fluids. *Acta Otolaryngologica*. 1970; 70: 58–61.
10. Silver, I, Li, ., Szalai, J, Johnston M. Relationship between intracranial pressure and cervical lymphatic pressure and flow rates in sheep. *American Journal of Physiology* 1999. 277,6–2:R1712–R1717.
11. Jones HC, Lopman BA. The relation between CSF pressure and ventricular dilatation in hydrocephalic HTx rats. *European Journal of Pediatric Surgery*. 1998, 8; S1: 55–58.
12. Cserr HF, Knopf PM. Cervical Lymphatics, the blood-brain barrier and immunoreactivity of the brain: a new view. *Immunology Today* 1992; 13: 507–512.
13. McComb JG, Davson H, Hyman S, Weiss MH. Cerebrospinal fluid drainage as influenced by ventricular pressure in the rabbit. *Journal of Neurosurgery* 1982; 56: 790–797.
14. Knopf PM, Cserr HF. Physiology and Immunology of lymphatic drainage of interstitial and cerebrospinal fluid from the brain. *Neuropathology and applied Neurobiology* 1995; 21: 175–180.
15. Koh L, Zakharov A, Johnston M. Integration of the subarachnoid space and lymphatics: Is it time to embrace a new concept of cerebrospinal fluid absorption? *Cerebrospinal Fluid Research* 2005, 2:6.
16. Bell GH, Emslie-Smith D, Paterson CR. 1980. *Textbook of Physiology*, 10th edition, Churchill Livingstone, Edinburgh, pp. 72 and 96.
17. Kinmonth JB. *The Lymphatics*, 2nd edition. Edward Arnold, London. pp 80. 1982.
18. Kinmonth JB. Some aspects of cardiovascular surgery. *Journal of the. Royal College of Surgeons Edinburgh* 1960; 5: 287–297.
19. Kinmonth JB. Sharpey-Schafer. Manometry of Human Thoracic Duct. *Journal of Physiology* 1959; 177: 41.
20. Browse NL. Response of lymphatics to sympathetic nerve stimulation. *Journal of Physiology* 1968; 19: 25.
21. Rogers S. *Tired or Toxic.* Syracuse, New York. Prestige Publishing 1990.
22. Lopachin RM, Aschner M. Glial-neuronal interactions: relevance to neurotoxic mechanisms. *Toxicology and Applied Pharmacology* 1993; 118: 141–158.
23. Iacono RF, Berria MI, Lascono EF. A triple staining procedure to evaluate phagocytic role of differentiated astrocytes. *Journal of Neuroscience Methods* 1991; 139: 225–230.
24. Morganti-Kossman MC, Kossman T, Wahl SM. Cytokines and Neuropathology. *Trends in Pharmaceutical Sciences* 1992; 13: 286–291.
25. Lindholm D, Castren E, Kiefer R, Zafra F, Thoenen H. Transforming growth factor-B1

in the rat brain; increase after injury and inhibition of astrocyte proliferation. *Journal of Cell Biology* 1992; 117: 395–400.

26. Sawada M, Suzumura A, Ohno K, Marunouchi T. Regulation of astrocyte proliferation by prostaglandin E2 and the a-subtype of protein kinase C. *Brain Research* 1993; 613: 67–73.
27. Perrin RN. Chronic fatigue syndrome: a review from the biomechanical perspective. *British Osteopathic Journal* 1993; 11: 15–23.
28. Perrin RN, Edwards J, Hartley P. An evaluation of the effectiveness of osteopathic treatment on symptoms associated with Myalgic Encephalomyelitis. A preliminary report. *Journal of Medical Engineering and Technology* 1998; 22, 1: 1–13.
29. Perrin RN. *The Involvement of Cerebrospinal Fluid and Lymphatic Drainage in Chronic Fatigue Syndrome/ME* (PhD Thesis). University of Salford, UK. 2005.
30. Perrin RN. Lymphatic drainage of the neuraxis and the CRI: a hypothetical model. *Journal of the American Osteopathic Association*. In press (accepted Jan 2007).

Chapter 2

1. Ramsay AM, O'Sullivan E. Encephalomyelitis simulating poliomyelitis. *Lancet* 1956; 270, 6926: 761–764.
2. Hutchinson A, Pinching L, Chambers T, Waterman J, Wayne N. (eds.). *A Report of the CFS/ME Working Group to the Chief Medical Officer* 2002.
3. Fukuda K, Straus SE, Hickie I, Sharpe MC, Dobbins JG, Komaroff A. The chronic fatigue syndrome: a comprehensive approach to its definition and study. International Chronic Fatigue Syndrome Study Group. *Annals of Internal Medicine* 1994; 121 (12): 953–959.
4. Sharpe M, Archard L, Banatvala J. A report: chronic fatigue syndrome: guidelines for research. *Journal of the Royal Society of Medicine* 1991; 84: 118–21.
5. Carruthers B. Definitions and aetiology of Myalgic Encephalomyelitis (ME): how the Canadian Consensus Clinical Definition of ME works. *Journal of Clinical Pathology* 2007; 60 (2): 117–119.
6. Da Costa JM. A Clinical Study of a Form of Functional Cardiac Disorder and its Consequences. *American Journal of Medical Science* 1871; 61: 17–52.
7. Lewis T. *The Soldiers Heart and the Effort Syndrome*. 1920 ; Paul B. Hober, New York.
8. Wesseley S, Chalder T, Hirsch S, Wallace P, Wright D. The Prevalence and Morbidity of chronic fatigue and chronic fatigue syndrome. A prospective primary care study. *American Journal of Public Health*. 1997; 87: 1449–1455.
9. Van Houdenhove B, Onghena P, Neerinckx E, Hellin J. 1995. Does High "Action-

Proneness" make People More Vulnerable to C.F.S.? A Controlled Psychometric Study. *Journal of Psychosomatic Research* 1995; 39 (5): 633–640.

10. Silver A, Haeney M, Vijayadurai P, Wilks D, Pattrick M, Main CJ. The Role of Fear of Physical Movement and Activity in Chronic Fatigue Syndrome. *Journal of Psychosomatic Research* 2002; 52, 6: 485–493.
11. Metzger FA, and Denney DR. Perception of cognitive performance in patients with chronic fatigue syndrome. *Annals Behavioural Medicine* 2002; 24(2): 106–12.
12 Fisher L, Chalder T. Childhood experiences of illness and parenting in adults with chronic fatigue syndrome. *Journal of Psychosomatic Research* 2003; 54 (5): 439–443.
13. McCrone P, Darbishire L, Ridsdale L, Seed P. The economic cost of chronic fatigue and chronic fatigue syndrome in UK primary care. *Psychological Medicine* 2003; 33 (2): 197–201.
14. Bierl C, Nisenbaum R, Hoaglin DC, Randall B, Jones AB, Unger ER, Reeves WC. Regional distribution of fatiguing illnesses in the United States: a pilot study. *Population Health Metr* 2004; 2: 1.
15. Pinching AJ. AIDS and CFS/ME: a tale of two syndromes. *Clinical Medicine* 2003; 3 (2): 188.
16. Naschitz JE, Sabo E, Dreyfuss D, Yeshurun D, Rosner I. 2003. The head-up tilt test in the diagnosis and management of chronic fatigue syndrome. *Israeli Medical Association Journal* 2003; 11: 807–11.
17. Lloyd AR., Broughton C, Dwyer J, Wakefield D. What is myalgic encephalomyelitis? *Lancet* 1988; 4; 1, 8597: 1286–7.
18. Gershon S, Shaw FH. Psychiatric sequelae of chronic exposure to organophosphorous insecticides. *Lancet* 1961; 1: 1371–1374.
19. Dunstan RH Donohoe M, Taylor W, Roberts TK, Murdoch RN, Watkins JA, McGregor NR. A preliminary investigation of chlorinated hydrocarbons and chronic fatigue syndrome. *Medical Journal of Australia* 1995; 163,6: 294–297.
20. Tahmaz N, Soutar A, Cherrie JW. Chronic fatigue and organophosphate pesticides in sheep farming: a retrospective study amongst people reporting to a UK pharmaco-vigilance scheme. *Annals of Occupational Hygiene* 2003; 47 (4): 261–7.
21. Rogers S. *Tired or Toxic*. Syracuse, New York. Prestige Publishing 1990.
22. Fiedler N, Kipen M, DeLuca J, Kelly- McNeil K, Natelson B. A controlled comparison of multiple chemical sensitivities and chronic fatigue syndrome. *Psychosomatic Medicine* 1996; 58: 38–49.
23. Buchwald D, Garrity D. Comparison of patients with chronic fatigue syndrome, fibromyalgia and multiple chemical sensitivities. *Archives of Internal Medicine* 1994; 154: 2049–2053.

24. Nawab SS, Miller CS, Dale JK, Greenberg BD, Friedman TC, Chrousos GP, Straus SE, Rosenthal NE. Self-reported sensitivity to chemical exposures in five clinical populations and healthy controls. *Psychiatry Research* 2000; 95, 1: 67–74.
25. Hickie I, Lloyd A, Wakefield D. Immunological and psychological dysfunction in patients receiving immunotherapy for chronic fatigue syndrome. Australia & New Zealand. *Journal of Psychiatry* 1992; 26, 2: 249–256.
26. Kerr JR et al 2006. Current research priorities in Chronic Fatigue Syndrome / Myalgic Encephalomyelitis (CFS/ME): disease mechanisms, a diagnostic test and specific treatments. *Journal Clinical Pathology* 2007; 60 (2): 113–116.
27. Harvey WT. A Flight Surgeon's Personal View of an Emerging Illness. *Aviat Space Environ* 1989; 60, 12: 1119–1201.
28. Simpson LO. Non-discocytic erythrocytes in myalgic encephalomyelitis. *New Zealand Medical Journal* 1989; 102: 126–7.
29. Spurgin M. The role of Blood Cell Morphology in the Pathogenesis of ME/CFIDS. *The CFIDS Chronicle* Summer 1995: 55–58.
30. Puri BK, Holmes J, Hamilton G. Eicosapentaenoic acid-rich essential fatty acid supplementation in chronic fatigue syndrome associated with symptom remission and structural brain changes. *International Journal of Clinical Practice* 2004; 58(3): 297–299.
31. Hokama Y, Uto GA, Palafox NA, Enlander D, Jordan E, Cocchetto A. 2003. Chronic Phase Lipids in Sera of Chronic Fatigue Syndrome, Chronic Ciguatera Fish Poisoning (CCFP), Hepatitis B, and Cancer with Antigenic Epitope Resembling Ciguatoxin, as Assessed with Mab-CTX. *Journal of Clinical and Laboratory Analysis* 2003; 17 (4): 132–139.
32. Smith S. Sullivan K. Examining the influence of biological and psychological factors on cognitive performance in chronic fatigue syndrome: a randomized, double-blind, placebo-controlled, crossover study. *International Journal of Behavioral Medicine* 2003; 10 (2): 162–173.
33. Hotopf A, David A, Hull L, Ismail K, Unwin C, Wesseley S. Role of vaccinations as risk factors for ill health in veterans of the Gulf War: cross sectional study. *British Medical Journal* 2000; 320: 1363–1367.
34. Shaheen S. Shots in the desert and Gulf War Syndrome. *British Medical Journal* 2000; 320: 1351–1352.

Chapter 3

1. Da Costa JM. A Clinical Study of a Form of Functional Cardiac Disorder and its Consequences. *American Journal of Medical Science* 1871; 61: 17–52.

2. Korr IM. The Spinal Cord as Organizer of Disease Processes: The Peripheral Autonomic Nervous System. *Journal of American Osteopathic Association* 1979; 79: 82–90.
3. Korr IM, (Ed.). *Sustained Sympatheticonia as a Factor in Disease: The Neurobiological Mechanism in Manipulative Therapy* 1978; Plenum, New York. pp. 229–268.
4. Korr IM, Buzzell H, Hix LE. The Sympathetic Nervous System as Mediator Between the Somatic and Supportive Process. In: Kugelmass IN (Ed.) *The Physiological Basis of Osteopathic Medicine* 1970; Indianapolis, American Academy of Osteopathy, 21–38.
5. Korr IM, Denslow JS, Krems AD. Quantitative Studies of Chronic Facilitation in Human Motoneuron Pools. *American Journal of Physiology* 1947; 150: 229–238.
6. Korr IM, Wright HM, Chase JA. Cutaneous Patterns of Sympathetic Activity in Clinical Abnormalities of the Musculoskeletal System. *Journal of Neural Transmission* 1964; 25: 589–606.
7. Dale HH, Gaddum JH. Reactions of denervated voluntary muscle, and their bearing on the mode of action of parasympathetic and related nerves. *Journal of Physiology* 1930; 70(2): 109–144.
8. Feldberg W, Gaddum JH. The chemical transmitter at synapses in a sympathetic ganglion *Journal of Physiology* 1934; 81(3): 305–319.
9. Bannister Sir R, and Mathias C, (Eds.). *Autonomic Failure*. 3rd edition, 1993; Oxford Medical, Oxford.
10. Vizi ES, Orso E, Osipenko ON, Hasko G, Elenkov IJ. Neurochemical, Electrophysiological and Immunocytochemical Evidence for a Noradrenergic Link Between the Sympathetic Nervous System and Thymocytes. *Neuroscience* 1995; 68 (4): 1263–1276.
11. Lewis T. *The Soldier's Heart and the Effort Syndrome*. 1920; Paul B. Hober: New York.
12. Ramsay AM, O'Sullivan E. Encephalomyelitis simulating poliomyelitis. *Lancet* 1956; 270 (6926): 761–764.
13. Hotchin NA, Read R, Smith DG, Crawford DH. Active Epstein-Barr virus infection in post-viral fatigue syndrome. *Journal of Infection* 1989; 18 (2): 143–50.
14. Richards AJ. Epstein-Barr virus and chronic fatigue syndrome. *Journal of Rheumatology* 1988; 15(10): 1595.
15. Jones JF. Epstein-Barr virus and the chronic fatigue syndrome: a short review. *Microbiological Science* 1988; 5(12): 366–369.
16. Nairn C, Galbraith DN, Clements GB. Comparison of Coxsackie B neutralisation and enteroviral PCR in chronic fatigue patients. *Journal of Medical Virology* 1995; 46(4): 310–313.

17. Soto NE, Straus SE. Chronic Fatigue Syndrome and Herpes viruses: the Fading Evidence. *Herpes* 2000; 7(2): 46–50.
18. Vladutiu GD, Natelson BH. Association of medically unexplained fatigue with ACE insertion/deletion polymorphism in Gulf War veterans. *Muscle Nerve* 2004; 30 (1):38–43.
19. Noguchi H, Kaname T, Sekimoto T, Senba K, Nagata Y, Araki M, Abe M, Nakagata N, Ono T, Yamamura K, Araki K. Naso-maxillary deformity due to frontonasal expression of human transthyretin gene in transgenic mice. *Genes Cells* 2002; 7 (10): 1087–98.
20. Chatel M, Menault F, Pecker J. Arguments in favor of the genetic origin of malformed syringohydromyelic pictures. *Neurochirurgie* 1979; 25 (3): 160–5.

Chapter 4

1. Georgiades E, Behan WM, Kilduff LP, Hadjicharalambous M, Mackie EE, Wilson J, Ward SA, Pitsiladis YP. Chronic Fatigue Syndrome: New Evidence for a Central Fatigue Disorder. *Clinical Science* 2003; 105 (2): 213–218.
2. Lerner AM, Beqaj SH, Deeter RG, Dworkin HJ, Zervos M, Chang CH, Fitzgerald JT, Goldstein J, O'Neill W. A six-month trial of valacyclovir in the Epstein-Barr virus subset of chronic fatigue syndrome: improvement in left ventricular function. Drugs Today. 2002; 38 (8): 549–561.
3. Agut H, Aubin JT. A new virus: the human herpes virus 6. *Rev Prat* 1994; 44: 7871–7874.
4. Blondel-Hill E, Shafran SD. Treatment of the chronic fatigue syndrome. A review and practical guide. *Drugs* 1993; 46 (4): 639–651.
5. Demettre E, Bastide L, D'Haese A, De Smet K, De Meirleir K, Tiev KP, Englebienne P, Lebleu B. Ribonuclease L proteolysis in peripheral blood mononuclear cells of chronic fatigue syndrome patients. *J Biol Chem* 2002; 277, 38: 35746–35751.
6. Snell CR, Vanness JM, Strayer DR, Stevens SR. Physical performance and prediction of 2-5A synthetase/Rnase L antiviral pathway activity in patients with chronic fatigue syndrome. *In Vivo* 2002; 16 (2): 107–109.
7. Suhadolnik RJ, Peterson DL, O'Brien K, Cheney PR, Herst CV, Reichenbach NL. Biochemical evidence for a novel low molecular weight 2-5A-dependent Rnase L in chronic fatigue syndrome. *J Interferon Cytokine Res* 1997; 17 (7): 377–385.
8. Pall ML, Satterlee JD. Elevated nitric oxide/peroxynitrite mechanism for the common etiology of multiple chemical sensitivity, chronic fatigue syndrome and posttraumatic stress disorder. *Ann NY Acad Science* 2001; 933: 323–329.
9. Pall ML. Elevated, sustained peroxynitrite levels as the cause of chronic fatigue syndrome. *Medical Hypotheses* 2000; 54 (1): 115–125.

10. Wakefield AJ, Puleston JM, Montgomery SM, Anthony A, O'Leary JJ, Murch SH. Review article: the concept of entero-colonic encephalopathy, autism and opioid receptor ligands. *Alimentary Pharmacology & Therapeutics* 2002; 16 (4): 663–674.
11. Levine PH, Peterson D, McNamee FL, O'Brien K, Gridley G, Hagerty M, Brady J, Fears T, Atherton M, Hoover R. Does Chronic Fatigue Syndrome Predispose to Non-Hodgkin's Lymphoma? *Cancer Research* 2002; 52 (19): 5516s-5518s; discussion 5518s-5521s.
12. Eby NL, Grufferman S, Flannelly CM, Schold SC Jr, Vogel FS, Burger PC. Increasing incidence of primary brain lymphoma in the US. *Cancer* 1988; 62 (11): 2461–2465.
13. Goldstein J. *Chronic Fatigue Syndromes: The Limbic Hypothesis*. 1993; The Haworth Medical Press, New York.
14. Schmaling KB, Lewis DH, Fiedelak JI, Mahurin R, Buchwald DS. Single-photon emission computerized tomography and neurocognitive function in patients with chronic fatigue syndrome. *Psychosomatic Medicine* 2003; 65(1): 129–136.
15. Nairn C, Galbraith DN, Clements GB. Comparison of Coxsackie B neutralisation and enteroviral PCR in chronic fatigue patients. *Journal of Medical Virology* 1995; 46(4): 310–3.
16. Lerner AM, Beqaj SH, Deeter RG, Dworkin HJ, Zervos M, Chang CH, Fitzgerald JT, Goldstein J, O'Neill W. A six-month trial of valacyclovir in the Epstein-Barr virus subset of chronic fatigue syndrome: improvement in left ventricular function. *Drugs Today* 2002; 38 (8): 549–561.
17. Straus SE, Dale JK, Tobi M, Lawley T, Preble O, Blaese RM, Hallahan C, Henle W. 1988. Acyclovir Treatment of the CF. Lack of Efficacy in a Placebo-controlled Trial. *New England Journal Medicine* 1988; 319 (26): 1692–1698.
18. Scott LV, Dinan TG. The neuroendocrinology of chronic fatigue syndrome: focus on the hypothalamic-pituitary-adrenal axis. *Funct Neurol* 1999; 14 (1): 3–11.
19. Kuratsune H, Yamaguti K, Sawada M, Kodate S, Machii T, Kanakura Y, Kitani T. Dehydroepiandrosterone sulfate deficiency in chronic fatigue syndrome. *International Journal of Molecular Medicine* 1998; 1 (1): 143–146.
20. Knook L, Kavelaars A, Sinnema G, Kuis W, Heijnen CJ. High nocturnal melatonin in adolescents with chronic fatigue syndrome. J Clin Endocrinol Metab. 2000; 85 (10): 3690–3692.
21. Shepherd C. *Living with M.E., the Chronic Post-viral Syndrome*. Vermilion Press, London; 1998.
22. Allain TJ, Bearn JA, Coskeran P, Jones J, Checkley A, Butler J, Wessely S, Miell JP. Changes in growth hormone, insulin, insulin-like growth factors (IGFs), and IGF-binding protein-1 in chronic fatigue syndrome. *Biological Psychiatry* 1997; 41 (5): 567–573.

23. Natelson BH, Cheu J, Pareja J, Ellis SP, Policastro T, Findley TW. Randomized, double blind, controlled placebo-phase in trial of low dose phenelzine in the chronic fatigue syndrome. Psychopharmacology. 1996; 124 (3): 226–230.
24. Vercoulen JH, Swanink CM, Zitman FG, Vreden SG, Hoofs MP, Fennis JF, Galama JM, van der Meer JW, Bleijenberg G. Randomised, double-blind, placebo-controlled study of fluoxetine in chronic fatigue syndrome. *Lancet* 1996; 347 (9005): 858–861.
25. Miller JB. Intradermal provocative-neutralizing food testing and subcutaneous food extract injection therapy. In: *Food Allergy and Intolerance* edited by Brostoff J and Challacombe SJ (Eds.). Baillieré Tindall, London; 1987.
26. Fell P, Brostoff J. A single dose desensitization for summer hay fever. Results of a double blind study. *European Journal of Clinical Pharmacology* 1990; 38 (1): 77–79.
27. Pall ML Elevated, sustained peroxynitrite levels as the cause of chronic fatigue syndrome. *Medical Hypotheses* 2000; 54 (1): 115–125.
28. Reichlin S. Neuroendocrine-immune interactions. *New England Journal of Medicine* 1993; 329 (17): 1246–1253.
29. Harman D. Aging: A theory based on free radical and radiation chemistry. *Gerontology* 1996; 11 (3): 298–300.
30. Kodama M, Kodama T, Murakami M. The value of the dehydroepiandrosterone-annexed vitamin C infusion treatment in the clinical control of chronic fatigue syndrome (CFS). II. Characterization of CFS patients with special reference to their response to a new vitamin C infusion treatment. *In Vivo* 1996; 10 (6): 585–596.

Chapter 5

1. Renfro L, Feder HM, Lane TJ, Manu P, Matthews DA. Yeast Connection Among 100 patients with Chronic Fatigue Syndrome. *American Journal of Medicine* 1989; 86: 165–168.
2. Mulder SJ. Bacteria of food and human intestine are the most possible sources of the gad-trigger of type 1 diabetes. *Medical Hypotheses* 2005; 65(2): 308–311.
3. Krop JJ. Treatment and prophylaxis for patients suffering from environmental hypersensitivity disorder. *Folia Med Cracov* 1993; 34(1–4): 159–172.
4. Simpson JW. Diet and large intestinal disease in dogs and cats. *Journal of Nutrition* 1998; 128(12 Suppl): 2717S-2722S.
5. Hasegawa M, Ohtomo M, Mita H, Akiyama K. Clinical aspects of patients with MCS – (from the standpoint of allergy). *Arerugi* 2005; 54(5): 478–484.
6. Morris DH, Stare FJ. Unproven diet therapies in the treatment of CFS. *Archives of Family Medicine* 1993; 2 (2): 181–186.

7. Heap LC, Peters TJ, Wessely S. Vitamin B status in patients with chronic fatigue syndrome. *Journal of the Royal Society of Medicine* 1999; 92 (4): 183–185.
8. Werbach M. Nutritional strategies for treating Chronic Fatigue Syndrome. *Alternative Medicine Review* 1998; 5: 93–108.
9. Cox IM, Campbell MJ, Dowson D. Red blood cell magnesium and chronic fatigue syndrome. *Lancet* 1991; 337 (8744): 757–60.
10. Russell IJ, Michalek JE, Flechas JD, Abraham GE. Treatment of fibromyalgia syndrome with Super Malic: a randomized, double blind, placebo controlled, crossover pilot study. *Journal of Rheumatology* 1995; 22 (5): 953–958.
11. Puri BK, Counsell SJ, Zaman R, Main J, Collins AG, Hajnal JV, Davey NJ. Relative increase in choline in the occipital cortex in chronic fatigue syndrome. *Acta Psychiatr Scand* 2002; 106: 224–226.
12. Crook WG. Candida colonization and allergic phenomena. *Hosp Pract* (official edition) 1994; 19 (9): 20.
13. Girois SB, Chapuis F, Decullier E, Revol BG. Adverse effects of antifungal therapies in invasive fungal infections: review and meta-analysis. *Eur J Clin Microbiol Infect Dis* 2006; 25(2): 138–149.
14. Friedberg F, Jason LA. Chronic fatigue syndrome and fibromyalgia: clinical assessment and treatment. *Journal of Clinical Psychology* 2001; 57 (4): 433.
15. Fulcher KY, White PD. Randomised Controlled Trial of Graded Exercise in Patients with the Chronic Fatigue syndrome. *British Medical Journal* 1997; 314: 1647–1652.
16. Paul L, Wood L, Behan WM, Maclaren WM. Demonstration of delayed recovery from fatiguing exercise in chronic fatigue syndrome. *European Journal of Neurology*. 1999; 6 (1): 63–69.
17. Reid S, Chalder T, Cleare A, Hotopf M, Wessely S. Chronic fatigue syndrome. *British Medical Journal* 2000; 320 (7230): 292–296.
18. Blenkiron P, Edwards R, Lynch S. Associations between perfectionism, mood, and fatigue in chronic fatigue syndrome: a pilot study. *J Nerv Ment Dis* 1997; 187 (9): 566–70.
19. Sharpe M. Chronic fatigue syndrome. *Psychiatric Clinics of North America* 1996; 19 (3): 549–573.
20. Sharpe M, Hawton K, Simkin S, Surawy C, Hackmann A, Klimes I, Peto T, Warrell D, Seagroatt V. Cognitive behaviour therapy for the chronic fatigue syndrome: a randomized controlled trial. *British Medical Journal* 1996; 312 (7022): 22–26.
21. Deale A, Chalder T, Marks I, Wessely S. Cognitive Behavioural Therapy for Chronic Fatigue Syndrome: A Randomised Controlled Trial. *British Medical Journal* 1996; 312: 22–26.

22. Lloyd AR, Hickie I, Brockman A, Hickie C, Wilson A, Dwyer J, Wakefield D. Immunologic and psychologic therapy for patients with chronic fatigue syndrome: a double-blind, placebo-controlled trial. *American Journal of Medicine* 1993; 94 (2): 197–203.
23. Lynch S, Seth R, Montgomery S. Antidepressant therapy in the chronic fatigue syndrome. *British Journal of General Practice* 1991; 41 (349): 339–342.
24. Wilson A, Hickie I, Lloyd A, Wakefield D. The treatment of chronic fatigue syndrome: science and speculation. *American Journal of Medicine* 1994; 96 (6): 544–550.
25. Klonoff DC. Chronic fatigue syndrome. *Clin Infect Dis* 1992; 15 (5): 812–823.
26. Gregg VH. Hypnosis in chronic fatigue syndrome. *Journal of the Royal Society of Medicine* 1997; 12: 682–683.
27. Korr IM. The Spinal Cord as Organizer of Disease Processes: The Peripheral Autonomic Nervous System. *Journal of American Osteopathic Association* 1979; 79: 82–90.
28. Korr IM, (Ed.). *Sustained Sympatheticonia as a Factor in Disease: the Neurobiological Mechanism in Manipulative Therapy*. Plenum, New York. 1978: pp. 229–268.
29. Korr IM. The Sympathetic Nervous System as Mediator Between the Somatic and Supportive Process. *The Physiological Basis of Osteopathic Medicine* 1970; 21–38.
30. Korr IM, Denslow JS, Krems AD. Quantitative Studies of Chronic Facilitation in Human Motor Neuron Pools. *American Journal of Physiology* 1947; 150: 229–238.
31. Korr IM, Wright HM, Chase JA. Cutaneous Patterns of Sympathetic Activity in Clinical Abnormalities of the Musculoskeletal System. *Journal of Neural Transmission* 1984; 25: 589–606.
32. Korr IM, Wright HM, Thomas PE. Effects of Experimental and Myofascial Insults on Cutaneous Patterns of Sympathetic Activity in Man. *Journal of Neural Transmission* 1962; 23 (22): 330–355.
33. Korr IM, Wright HM, Thomas PE. 1960. Local & Regional Variations in Cutaneous Vasomotor Tone of the Human Trunk. *Journal of Neural Transmission* 1960; 22, 3: 34–52.

Chapter 6

1. Merton PA, Marsden CD, Morton HB. Is the Human Stretch Reflex Cortical Rather Than Spinal? *Lancet* 1973; 1 (7806): 759–761.
2. Puri BK, Counsell SJ, Zaman R, Main J, Collins AG, Hajnal JV, Davey NJ. Relative increase in choline in the occipital cortex in chronic fatigue syndrome. *Acta Psychiatr Scand* 2002; 106: 224–226.

3. Hoh D. Spine, and Skull surgery may help many with CFIDS, FMS: Chiari-malformation or cervical stenosis may be common in CFIDS & Fibromyalgia. *The CFIDS Chronicle* 1999; May/June, 10–12.

Chapter 7

1. Johnson WG, Hodge SE, Duvoisin R. Twin Studies and the genetics of Parkinson's disease: a reappraisal. *Movement Disorders* 1990; 5: 187–194.
2. Calne DB, Hochburg FH, Snow BJ, Nygaard T. Theories of Neurodegenerative Diseases: An Overview. *Annals of the NY Academy of Sciences* 1992; 648: 1–5.
3. Veronesi B. The use of cell cultures for evaluating neurotoxicity. In: *Neurotoxicology* Edited by Tilson HA and Mitchell CL. Raven Press, New York. 1992; pp. 21–49.
4. Tilson HA, Mitchell CL. *Neurotoxicology*. Raven Press, New York, 1992.
5. Sabljic A. 1991. Chemical topology and ecotoxicology. Sci Total Environ. Dec; 109–110: 197–220.
6. Perrin RN. The Involvement of Cerebrospinal Fluid and Lymphatic Drainage in Chronic Fatigue Syndrome/ME (PhD Thesis). University of Salford, UK. 2005.
7. Zhang JJ, Lioy PJ. Human exposure assessment in air pollution systems. *Scientific World Journal* 2002; 2: 497–513.
8. Morrell S, Kerr C, Driscoll T, Taylor R, Salkeld G, Corbett S. Best estimate of the magnitude of mortality due to occupational exposure to hazardous substances. *Occup Environ Med* 1998; 55(9): 634–641
9. Banerjee BD, Koner BC, Ray A. Immunotoxicity of pesticides: perspectives and trends. *Indian Journal of Experimental Biology* 1996; 34(8): 723–33
10. Wallace LA, Pellizzari E, Hartwell T, Rosenzweig M, Erickson M, Sparacino C, Zelon H. Personal exposure to volatile organic compounds. I. Direct measurements in breathing-zone air, drinking water, food, and exhaled breath. *Environmental Research* 1984; 35 (1): 293–319.
11. Agency for Toxic Substances and Disease Registry ATSDR- ToxFAQs. Sept 2005. http://www.atsdr.cdc.gov/tfacts3.html
12. Agency for Toxic Substances and Disease Registry ATSDR- ToxFAQs. Sept 2007. http://www.atsdr.cdc.gov/tfacts6.html
13. Hoet P, et al. 1997 Epidemic of liver disease caused by hydrochlorofluorocarbons used as ozone-sparing substitutes of chlorofluorocarbons *Lancet* 1997; 350 (9077): 556–559
14. Carpenter DO. Polychlorinated biphenyls (PCBs): routes of exposure and effects on human health. *Rev Environ Health* 2006; 21(1): 1–23.
15. Gotohda T, Tokunaga I, Kubo S, Morita K, Kitamura O, Eguchi A. Effect of toluene

inhalation on astrocytes and neurotrophic factor in rat brain. *Forensic Sci Int*. 2000; 113 (1–3): 233–238

16. Jovanovic JM, Jovanovic MM, Spasic MJ, Lukic SR.2004.Peripheral nerve conduction study in workers exposed to a mixture of organic solvents in paint and lacquer industry. *Croat Med J* 2004; 45 (6): 769–774
17. Sebastian A, Pehrson C, Larsson L. Elevated concentrations of endotoxin in indoor air due to cigarette smoking. *J Environ Monit* 2006; 8 (5): 519–22. Epub 2006 Mar 27
18. Lau K, McLean WG, Williams DP, Howard CV. Synergistic interactions between commonly used food additives in a developmental neurotoxicity test. *Toxicological Science* 2006; 90(1): 178–87. Epub 2005 Dec 13
19. Latinwo LM, Badisa VL, Ikediobi CO, CO, Lambert, Badisa RB. Effect of cadmium-induced oxidative stress on antioxidative enzymes in mitochondria and cytoplasm of CRL-1439 rat liver cells. *Int J Mol Med* 2006; 18 (3): 477–81.
20. Reed A, Dzon L, Loganathan BG, Whalen MM. Immunomodulation of human natural killer cell cytotoxic function by organochlorine pesticides. *Hum Exp Toxicol* 2004; 23(10): 463–471.
21. Weiss B. Neurobehavioural toxicity as a basis for risk assessment. *Trends in Pharmaceutical Science* 1988; 9: 59–62.
22. Needleman HL, Schell A, Bellinger D, Leviton A, Allred EN. The long-term exposure to low doses of lead in children. An 11–year follow-up report. *New England Journal of Medicine* 1990; 322: 83–88.
23. Drasch G, Aigner S, Roider G, Staiger F, Lipowsky G. Mercury in human colostrum and early breast milk. Its dependence on dental amalgam and other factors. *J Trace Elem Med Biol* 1998; 12 (1): 232–237.
24. Mutter J, Naumann J, Sadaghiani C, Walach H, Drasch G. Amalgam studies: disregarding basic principles of mercury toxicity. *Int J Hyg Environ Health* 2004; 207 (4): 391–397.
25. Lloyd AR., Broughton C, Dwyer J, Wakefield D. 1988. What is myalgic encephalomyelitis? *Lancet* 1988; 1 (8597): 1286–1287.
26. Garrel C, Lafond JL, Guiraud P, Faure P, Favier A. Induction of production of nitric oxide in microglial cells by insoluble form of aluminium. *Annals of the New York Academy of Science* 1994; 738: 455–461.
27. Gershon S, Shaw FH. Psychiatric sequelae of chronic exposure to organophosphorus insecticides. *Lancet* 1961; 1: 1371–1374.
28. Dunstan RH Donohoe M, Taylor W, Roberts TK, Murdoch RN, Watkins JA, McGregor NR. A preliminary investigation of chlorinated hydrocarbons and chronic fatigue syndrome. *Medical Journal of Australia* 1995; 163 (6): 294–297.

29. Croquet V., et al. 1,1, 1–trichloroethane-induced chronic active hepatitis. *Gastroenterol Clin Biol* 2003; 27 (1): 120–122.
30. Wallace L, Pellizzari E, Hartwell T, Zelon H, Sparacino C, Perritt R, Whitmore R. Concentrations of 20 volatile organic compounds in the air and drinking water of 350 residents of New Jersey compared with concentrations in their exhaled breath. *Journal of Occupational Medicine* 1986; 28 (8): 603–608.
31. Hardell L, Hallquist A, Mild KH, Carlberg M, Pahlson A, Lilja A. Cellular and cordless telephones and the risk for brain tumours. *European Journal of Cancer Prevention* 2002; 11 (4): 377–386.
32. Leszczynski D. Mobile Phones, Precautionary principle and future research. Letter; *Lancet* 2001; 358 (9294): 1733.
33. Hotopf A, David A, Hull L, Ismail K, Unwin C, Wessley S. Role of vaccinations as risk factors for ill health in veterans of the Gulf War: cross sectional study. *British Medical Journal* 2000;320: 1363–1367.
34. Shaheen S. Shots in the desert and Gulf War Syndrome. *British Medical Journal* 2000; 320: 1351–1352.
35. Hooper M. The Most Toxic War in Western Military History. Evidence submitted to the House of Commons Select Defence Committee. *7th Report of Defence Select Committee*: Gulf Veteran's Illnesses 1999.
36. Nicolson GL. Chronic infections as a common etiology for many patients with Chronic Fatigue Syndrome, Fibromyalgia Syndrome, and Gulf War Illnesses. *International Journal of Medicine* 1998; 1: 42–46.
37. Haley RW, Kurt TL. Self-reported Exposure to Neurotoxic Chemical Combinations in the Gulf War: A Cross-sectional Epidemiologic Study. *JAMA* 1997; 277: 231–237.
38. Hooper M, 2003, posted at http://osiris.sunderland.ac.uk/autism.
39. Fukuda K, Straus SE, Hickie I, Sharpe MC, Dobbins JG, Komaroff A. The chronic fatigue syndrome: a comprehensive approach to its definition and study. International Chronic Fatigue Syndrome Study Group. *Annals of Internal Medicine* 1994; 121 (12): 953–959.
40. Ismail K, Everitt B, Blatchley N, Hull L, Unwin C, David A, Wessley S. Is there a Gulf War syndrome? *Lancet* 1999; 353 (9148): 179–182.
41. Hyams KC, Wignall FS, Roswell R. War syndromes and their evaluation from the US civil war to the Persian Gulf War. *Annals of Internal Medicine* 1996; 125: 398–405.
42. Rogers S. *Tired or Toxic*. Syracuse, New York; Prestige Publishing 1990.
43. Hanin I. The Gulf War, stress and a leaky blood-brain barrier. *Nature Medicine* 1996; 12: 1307–1308.
44. Spence A. Khan F, Belch JJF. Enhanced sensitivity of the peripheral cholinergic vascular

response in patients with Chronic Fatigue Syndrome. *American Journal of Medicine* 2000; 108: 736–739.
45. Puri BK, Counsell SJ, Zaman R, Main J, Collins AG, Hajnal JV, Davey NJ. Relative increase in choline in the occipital cortex in chronic fatigue syndrome. *Acta psychiatr Scand* 2002; 106: 224–226.
46. Witte ST, Will LA, Olsen CR, Kinker JA, Miller-Graber P. Chronic selenosis in horses fed locally produced alfalfa hay. *Journal of the American Veterinary Medical Association* 1993; 1202 (3): 406–409.
47. Schwarz B, Salak N, Hofstotter H, Pajik W, Knotzer H, Mayr A, Hasibeder W. Intestinal ischemic reperfusion syndrome: pathophysiology, clinical significance, therapy. *Wien Klin Wochenschr* 1990; 111 (14): 539–548.
48. White JF. Intestinal pathophysiology in autism. *Exp Biol Med* 2003; 228 (6): 639–649.
49. Burke V, Gracey M. Effects of salicylate on intestinal absorption: in vitro and in vivo studies with enterotoxigenic micro-organisms. *Gut* 1980; 21 (8): 683–688.
50. Schumann K. Safety aspects of iron in food. *Ann Nutr Metab* 2001; 45 (3): 91–101.
51. Jett DA, Kuhlmann AC, Farmer SJ, Guilarte TR. Age-dependent effects of developmental lead exposure on performance in the Morris water maze. *Pharmacol Biochem Behav* 1997; 57 (1–2): 271–279.
52. Offit K, Groeger E, Turner S, Wadsworth EA, Weiser MA. The "duty to warn" a patient's family members about hereditary disease risks. *JAMA* 2004; 292 (12): 1469–1473.
53. Tilson HA, Mitchell CL. *Neurotoxicology*. Raven Press, New York; 1992.
54. Kammuller ME, Bloksma N, Seinen W, (eds) *Autoimmunity and Toxicology: immune disregulation induced by drugs and chemicals*. Elsevier, Amsterdam, 1989.
55. Czaja AJ, Donaldson PT. Genetic susceptibilities for immune expression and liver cell injury in autoimmune hepatitis. *Immunol Rev* 2000; 174: 250–259.

Chapter 8

1. Perrin RN. Chronic fatigue syndrome: a review from the biomechanical perspective. *British Osteopathic Journal* 1993; 11: 15–23.
2. Perrin RN, Edwards J, Hartley P. An evaluation of the effectiveness of osteopathic treatment on symptoms associated with Myalgic Encephalomyelitis. A preliminary report. *Journal of Medical Engineering and Technology* 1998; 22 (1): 1–13.
3. Keenan P. Brain MRI abnormalities exist in chronic fatigue syndrome (Editorial). *Journal of Neurological Sciences* 1999; 171: 1–2.
4. Lange G, Deluca J, Maldjian JA, Lee H, Tiersky LA, Natelson BH. Brain MRI

abnormalities exist in a subset of patients with chronic fatigue syndrome. *Journal of Neurological Sciences* 1999; 171 (1): 3–7.

5. Costa DC, Brostoff J, Tannock C. 1995. Brainstem Spect Studies in Normals, ME/CFS and Depression. *Nucl Med Commun* 1995; 15: 252–253.
6. Farrell M, Richards JG. Analysis of the reliability and validity of the kinetic communicator exercise device. *Med Sci Sports Exer* 1986; 18 (1): 44–49.
7. Hutchinson A, Pinching L, Chambers T, Waterman J, Wayne N. (eds.). A Report of the CFS/ME Working Group to the Chief Medical Officer. HMG, 2002.
8. Fukuda K, Straus SE, Hickie I, Sharpe MC, Dobbins JG, Komaroff A. The chronic fatigue syndrome: a comprehensive approach to its definition and study. International Chronic Fatigue Syndrome Study Group. *Annals of Internal Medicine* 1994; 121 (12): 953–959.
9. Sharpe M, Archard L, Banatvala J. 1991. A report: chronic fatigue syndrome: guidelines for research. *Journal of the Royal Society of Medicine* 1991; 84:118–121.
10. Carruthers B. Definitions and aetiology of Myalgic Encephalomyelitis (ME): how the Canadian Consensus Clinical Definition of ME works. *Journal of Clinical Pathology* 2007; 60 (2): 117–119.
11. Gasser HS. Properties of dorsal root unmedullated fibres on the two sides of the ganglion. *Journal of General Physiology* 1955; 38: 709–728.
12. Kinmonth JB. *The Lymphatics*, 2nd edition. London: Edward Arnold; 1982; 80.
13. Kinmonth JB. Some aspects of cardiovascular surgery. *Journal of the Royal College of Surgeons of Edinburgh* 1960; 5: 287–297.
14. Kinmonth JB. Sharpey-Schafer. Manometry of Human Thoracic Duct. *Journal of Physiology* 1959; 177: 41.
15. Vodder E. *Le drainage lymphatique, une nouvelle méthode thérapeutique*. Paris, France: Santé Pour Tous; 1936.
16. Browse NL. Response of lymphatics to sympathetic nerve stimulation. *Journal of Physiology* 1968; 19: 25.
17. Still AT. *Philosophy of Osteopathy*. Published by the Author, Kirksville, Mo. 1899.
18. Still AT. *The Philosophy and Mechanical Principles of Osteopathy* Kansas City USA: Hudson-Kimberly; 1902: 47.
19. Sutherland WG. *The Cranial Bowl* Mankato, Minnesota: Free Press Company; 1939.
20. Wales AL. (ed). Sutherland WG. *Teachings in the Science of Osteopathy*. Sutherland Cranial Teaching Foundation, Fort Worth, Texas; 1990.
21. Perrin RN. Lymphatic drainage of the neuraxis and the CRI: a hypothetical model. *Journal of the American Osteopathic Association*. In press (accepted Jan 2007).

Chapter 9

1. Webster GV. *Sage Sayings of Still*. Wetzel Publishing Co, London; 1928: 11.
2. 2. Sutherland WG. In: Wales AL (ed) *Teachings in the Science of Osteopathy*, Sutherland Cranial Teaching Foundation, Ft Worth, Texas; 1990: 64
3. Still AT. *The Philosophy and Mechanical Principles of Osteopathy*, Hudson-Kimberly, Kansas City, Mo; 1902: 68.
4. Still AT. *The Philosophy and Mechanical Principles of Osteopathy*, Hudson-Kimberly, Kansas City, Mo; 1902: 66.
5. Still AT. *The Philosophy and Mechanical Principles of Osteopathy*, Hudson-Kimberly, Kansas City, Mo; 1902: 150.
6. Woods JM, Woods RH. A physical finding relating to psychiatric disorders. *Journal of the American Osteopathic Association* 1961; 60: 988-993.
7. King HH, Lay EM. Osteopathy in the cranial field. In: Ward RC, ed. *Foundations for Osteopathic Medicine*. 2nd ed. Baltimore, Md: Lippincott Williams & Wilkins; 2003: 985 -1001.
8. Magoun HI. *Osteopathy in the Cranial Field*. 2nd ed. Kirksville, Mo: The Journal Printing Company; 1966.
9. Upledger JE, Vredevoogd JD. *Craniosacral Therapy*. Chicago, Ill: Eastland Press; 1983.
10. Nelson KE, Sergueef N, Glonek T. Recording the rate of the cranial rhythmic impulse. *Journal of the American Osteopathic Association*. 2006; 106 (6): 337-341.
11. .Norton JM, Sibley G, Broder-Oldach R. Characterization of the cranial rhythmic impulse in healthy human adults. *American Academy of Osteopathy Journal*. 1992; 2 (9):12, 26.
12. McAdoo J, Kuchera ML. Reliability of cranial rhythmic impulse palpation. *Journal of the American Osteopathic Association*. 1995; 95: 491.
13. Hanten WP, Dawson DD, Iwata M, Seiden M, Whitten FG, Zink T. Craniosacral rhythm: reliability and relationships with cardiac and respiratory rates. *J Orthop Sports Phys Ther*.1998; 27: 213 -218.
14. Perrin RN. The Involvement of Cerebrospinal Fluid and Lymphatic Drainage in Chronic Fatigue Syndrome/ME (PhD Thesis). University of Salford, UK, 2005.
15. Perrin RN. Lymphatic drainage of the neuraxis and the CRI: a hypothetical model. *Journal of the American Osteopathic Association*. Accepted Feb 2007: In Press.
16. Still AT. *Philosophy of Osteopathy*, Published by the Author, Kirksville, Mo; 1899: 197.

Chapter 10

1. Hartman L. *Handbook of Osteopathic Technique*. NMK Publishers. Herts; 1983.
2. Stoddard A. *Manual of Osteopathic Technique*. 3rd edition. Hutchinson, London, 1982.
3. Sutherland WG. *The Cranial Bowl*. Mankato, Minnesota, US: Free Press Company; 1939.
4. Sutherland WG. In: Wales AL (ed) *Teachings in the Science of Osteopathy*. Sutherland Cranial Teaching Foundation, Fort Worth, Texas, US; 1990.
5. Saidi G, Haines L. The management of children with chronic fatigue syndrome-like illness in primary care: a cross-sectional study. *British Journal of General Practice* 2006; 56(522): 43–47.

Chapter 11

1. Harlow BL, Signorello LB, Hall JE, Dailey C, Komaroff AL. Reproductive correlates of chronic fatigue syndrome. *American Journal of Medicine* 1998; 105(3A): 94S-99S.
2. Perrin RN. The Involvement of Cerebrospinal Fluid and Lymphatic Drainage in Chronic Fatigue Syndrome/ME (PhD Thesis). University of Salford, UK. 2005.
3. Hoh D. Skull surgery may help many with CFIDS, FMS: Chiari malformation or cervical stenosis may be common in CFIDS & Fibromyalgia. *The CFIDS Chronicle*, 1999 May/June, 10–12.
4. Cserr HF, Knopf PM. Cervical Lymphatics, the blood-brain barrier and immunoreactivity of the brain: a new view. *Immunology Today* 1992; 13: 507–512.
5. Devanur LD, Kerr JR. 2006. Chronic fatigue syndrome. *Journal of Clinical Virology* 2006; 37 (3): 139–150.
6. Gaab J, Rohleder N, Heitz V, Engert V, Schad T, Schurmeyer TH, Ehlert U. Stress-induced changes in LPS-induced pro-inflammatory cytokine production in chronic fatigue syndrome. *Psychoneuroendocrinology* 2005; 30 (2): 188–198
7. Browse NL. Response of lymphatics to sympathetic nerve stimulation. *Journal of Physiology* 1968; 19: 25.
8. King HH, Lay EM. Osteopathy in the cranial field. In: Ward RC (ed.) *Foundations for Osteopathic Medicine*. 2nd ed. Baltimore, Maryland, US: Lippincott Williams & Wilkins; 2003: 985–1001.
9. Still AT. *Philosophy of Osteopathy*. Published by the Author, Kirksville, Mo, US. 1899.
10. Sutherland WG. In: Wales AL (ed) *Teachings in the Science of Osteopathy*. Sutherland Cranial Teaching Foundation, Ft Worth, Texas, US; 1990.

11. Perrin RN, Edwards J, Hartley P. An evaluation of the effectiveness of osteopathic treatment on symptoms associated with Myalgic Encephalomyelitis. A preliminary report. *Journal of Medical Engineering and Technology* 1998; 22 (1): 1–13.
12. Stejskal VD et al. Metal-specific lymphocytes: biomarkers of sensitivity in man. *Neuro Endocrinol Letters* 1999; 20 (5): 289–298.
13. Genuis SJ, Genuis SK. Human exposure assessment and relief from neuropsychiatric symptoms: case study of a hairdresser. *J Am Board FAM Pract* 2004; 17 (2): 136–141.
14. Racciatti D, Vecchiet J,Ceccomancini A,Ricci F, Pizzigallo E. Chronic fatigue syndrome following a toxic exposure. *Sci Total Environ* 2001; 270 (1–3): 27–31.

Useful names and addresses

CFS/ME

Organisations in the UK

Action for ME
Action for ME is a UK charity working to improve the lives of people with ME. They campaign for more research, better services and treatments.
PO Box 1302
Wells,
Somerset,
BA5 1YE, UK
Tel: 01749 670799
Website: www.afme.org.uk

AYME (Association of Young People with ME)
PO Box 5766
Milton Keynes
MK10 1AQ, UK
Tel: 08451 23 23 89
Email: info@ayme.org.uk
Website: www.ayme.org.uk

FORME (Fund for Osteopathic Research into ME)
FORME is dedicated to helping osteopathic research into chronic fatigue syndrome (CFS/ME). FORME has funded research that has led to the scientific support of The Perrin Technique™ and aims to support further projects looking into the physical nature of CFS/ME. One of its main aims is to disseminate the findings of Dr Perrin's continuing research.
Registered Office:
83 Whittaker Lane,
Prestwich,
Manchester M25 1ET, UK
Website: www.forme-cfs.co.uk

Invest In M.E.
Invest in ME was set up in the UK with the objective of making a change in how ME is treated in the press and by the Government's Department of Health.
Tel: 02392 252365
Website: www.investinme.org

ME Association
The ME Association (MEA), founded in 1976, funds and supports research and provides information and advice, education and training in the field of CFS/ME. It aims to avoid duplicating the work undertaken by other voluntary and statutory agencies.
4 Corringham Road
Stanford le Hope
Essex SS17 0AH, UK
Tel: 01375 642466
Website: www.meassociation.org.uk (This useful site has listings of local societies throughout the world.)

(MERGE) ME Research UK
ME Research UK is based in Dundee, and holds the database on all research into ME in archive form.
ME Research UK
The Gateway
North Methven Street
Perth PH1 5PP, UK

Telephone/Fax: 01738 451234
E-mail: meruk@pkavs.org.uk
Website: www.meresearch.org.uk

Australia

ME Society of New South Wales
www.me-cfs.org.au

ME/Chronic Fatigue Syndrome Society of Victoria
http://avoca.vicnet.net.au/~mecfs

CFS Support
CFS Support is a site for people wishing to find local support groups.
Email: CfsSupport@aapt.net.au
Website: http://cfssupport.netfirms.com

Canada

ME Canada
246 Queen Street
Suite 400
Ottawa
Ontario
K1P 5E4
Canada
Tel: (613) 563 7514
Fax: (613) 567-0614
E-mail: info@mecan.ca
Website: www.mecan.ca

Ireland

Irish ME Trust
Carmichael House
North Brunswick Street
Dublin 7, Eire
Tel: 1890 200 912

Int. tel: 00 353 1 401 3629
Int. fax: 00 353 1 401 3736
E-mail: info@imet.ie
Website: www.imet.ie

New Zealand

ANZMES
PO Box 36 307
Northcote
Auckland 1309
New Zealand
Website: http://www.anzmes.org.nz

South Africa

MEASA (ME Association of South Africa)
PO Box 1802
Umhlanga Rocks
4320
Kwa Zulu Natal
South Africa
Email: arl@mweb.co.za

USA

CFIDS Association
The CFIDS Association of America is the nation's leading charitable organization dedicated to conquering chronic fatigue and immune dysfunction syndrome.
PO Box 220398
Charlotte
NC 28222-0389
USA
Tel: 00 1 800 442 3437 (toll free in the USA)
Website: www.cfids.org

The NCF (The National CFIDS Foundation)
The NCF is a national non-profit organisation that funds research and provides information, education, and support to people who have chronic fatigue syndrome.

103 Aletha Road
Needham
MA 02192
USA
Tel: 00 1 781 449 3535
Website: www.ncf-net.org

Other countries

CFS/ME is universal and there are many countries with national CFS/ME patient support groups. They can usually be found by searching on the worldwide web. Alas, there are many more countries where the sufferer does not have any official representation or recognition of the existence of the disease. Hopefully, this publication can be used to help lobby the relevant authorities in showing that CFS/ME is a real physical entity and should be researched and recognised.

OSTEOPATHY

GOsC (General Osteopathic Council)
General Osteopathic Council
176 Tower Bridge Road
London, SE1 3LU, UK
Tel: +44 (0) 207 357 6655
Fax: +44 (0) 207 357 0011
Email info@osteopathy.org.uk
Website: www.osteopathy.org.uk

AOA (American Osteopathic Association)
AOA also provides health information to patients and media interested in osteopathic medicine.

Chicago Office (Headquarters):
142 East Ontario Street
Chicago, IL 60611, USA
Toll-free phone: (800) 621-1773
General phone: (312) 202-8000
Fax (312) 202-8200

Washington Office:
1090 Vermont Ave. NW
Suite 510
Washington, DC 20005
Toll-free phone: (800) 962-9008
General phone: (202) 414-0140
Fax: (202) 544-3525
Website: www.osteopathic.org

CHIROPRACTIC

GCC (General Chiropractic Council)
44 Wicklow Street, London,
WC1X 9HL, UK
Tel: +44 (0) 20 7713 5155
Fax: +44 (0) 20 7713 5844
Email enquiries@gcc-uk.org
Website: www.gcc-uk.org

American Chiropractic Association
1701 Clarendon Boulevard
Arlington, VA 22209, USA
Fax: (703) 243 2593

PHYSIOTHERAPY

CSP (The Chartered Society of Physiotherapy)
The Chartered Society of Physiotherapy
14 Bedford Row
London, WC1R 4ED, UK
Telephone: 020 7306 6666
Fax: 020 7306 6611
Textphone: 020 7314 7890
Email: enquiries@csp.org.uk
Website: www.csp.org.uk

American Physical Therapy Association
1111 North Fairfax Street
Alexandria, VA 22314–1488, USA
Tel: (703) 684 APTA (2782) or 800/999-APTA (2782)
TDD: (703) 683 6748
Fax: (703) 684 7343
Website: www.apta.org

Glossary

A

ABDOMEN: The lower part of the trunk that lies between the thorax and the pelvis. The abdominal cavity contains the stomach and intestines, plus other internal organs and glands, e.g. the liver and pancreas.

ACUPUNCTURE: The puncture of the body by one or more needles to relieve pain, induce anaesthesia, and improve the health of a person. It is based on the Chinese philosophy of Tch'I (the energy of life) that is a balance of the positive Yin and the negative Yang. The acupuncture takes place along meridians, which are pathways of energy under the skin. The flow of energy is obstructed in disease states. By inserting a gold, copper or silver needle into a blocked meridian, the flow of energy is improved.

ACETYLCHOLINE: One of the substances that aids the transmission of impulses from one nerve to another, and from a nerve to its target organ.

ACID: A substance that forms hydrogen ions in solution, and combines with an alkaline material to form a salt. Acids have a pH value of less than 7.

ACYCLOVIR: A drug used against viruses. It is known to be helpful in the treatment of herpes infections.

ADRENALINE (or epinephrine): A hormone secreted by the adrenal gland. It stimulates the sympathetic nervous system. It is also manufactured synthetically, and used for its stimulating properties.

ADRENERGIC RECEPTORS: The places in the body on which adrenaline and equivalent chemicals (e.g. noradrenaline) exert their stimulant action on the sympathetic nervous system.

ADRENO-MEDDULLARY: Pertaining to or arising from the medulla of the adrenal gland.

AETIOLOGY: The cause of a disorder.

AGRANULAR: Not consisting of granules or grains.

ALBICANS: White.

ALKALI: A compound that forms a salt when mixed with an acid. Alkalis possess a pH value of more than 7.

AMPHETAMINE: A powerful and addictive drug which has a similar effect to adrenaline, and stimulates the sympathetic nervous system.

ANAEMIA (U.S. anemia): The condition that arises when the red blood cell and/or haemoglobin count falls below the normal level.

ANATOMICAL: Pertaining to the body's structure.

ANATOMY: The science dealing with the structure of the human and animal body.

ANTAGONIST: A substance that neutralises the action of another; a muscle that counteracts the action of another muscle (its agonist).

ANTERIOR: In front of; at the front.

ANTERIOR HORN CELL: A horn-shaped region found in the front part of the spinal cord.

ANTERO-LATERAL: Positioned towards the front and outside of a structure.

ANTIBODIES: Substances in the blood that fight against different toxins or foreign bodies (known as antigens).

ANTIDEPRESSANTS: The collective name given to those drugs that prevent or relieve depression.

ANTIVIRAL: Working against viruses.

AROMATHERAPY: The treatment of certain disorders by the use of aromatic, essential oils during massage.

ARTERY: A tube or vessel that conveys blood from the heart to the rest of the body.

ARTHRITIS: Inflammation of a joint, due to either a disease or the process of wear and tear.

AUSCULTATION: Listening for certain sounds within the body by using either the ear or a stethoscope.

AUTONOMIC: Not under voluntary control.

AUTONOMIC NERVOUS SYSTEM: A section of the nervous system that regulates the systems of the body that are not under voluntary control.

B

BRONCHUS: One of the larger tubes through which air passes from the windpipe to the smaller bronchioles within the lungs.

BUFFER: A chemical system that prevents change in the concentration of other chemical substances. Usually to keep acid/alkali levels in equilibrium.

C

CANDIDA: Yeast-like fungi that naturally occur in a healthy body but are capable of causing disease.

CANDIDIASIS: Infection caused by Candida.

CANTHUS: Part of the facial bone to the side of the eye.

CARBONIC ACID: A solution of carbon dioxide and water.

CARDIAC: Pertaining to the heart.

CARDIOLOGIST: A heart specialist.

CARDIOVASCULAR SYSTEM: The system composed of the heart and the blood vessels.

CEREBROSPINAL FLUID: The fluid surrounding and bathing the brain and the spinal cord.

CERVICAL: Pertaining to the neck.

CHOLINERGIC: The nerves that release the transmitter substance acetylcholine; an agent that stimulates the release of acetylcholine.

CHRONIC: Long lasting.

COCCYX: The triangular bone at the tail-end of the spine formed by the fusion of 3-5 vertebrae.

CONTRACTILE: Possessing the ability to contract, e.g. muscle.

CONTRACTION: A shortening (pulling together) of tissue.

CORTEX: The outer layer of a structure.

CRANIAL: Pertaining to the skeleton of the head (the cranium).

CRANIO-SACRAL: Pertaining to the cranium and the sacrum. Used mostly in relation to the rhythm of the CFS/ME, which travels from the head to the sacrum at the base of the spine.

D

DECEREBRATE: Stopping the function of the cerebrum (the main portion of the brain) by severing the brain stem, or by cutting off the blood supply to the brain.

DIAGNOSIS: Determining the type and exact nature of a disease.

DIATETIC: Pertaining to the diet for health purposes.

DILATION: The act of expanding.

DISC (DISK): A flat, thin, circular structure. Intervertebral discs contain fibrous outer layers surrounding soft, jelly-like centres. They lie between the bodies of adjacent vertebrae in the spinal column and act as shock absorbers.

DISTAL: At the further end.

DORSAL: Pertaining to the back; positioned on the back surface; Another name for thoracic, e.g., the dorsal spine.

DYSFUNCTION: An impairment or abnormality in the functioning of an organ or system in the body.

E

ELECTRON MICROSCOPY: Examination with a microscope that emits a beam of electrons (negatively charged particles of an atom). This beam forms an image for viewing on a fluorescent screen.

EPIDEMIC: The term given to an outbreak of a disease that affects a large number of people in the same location, and at the same time.

EPSTEIN-BARR VIRUS: A herpes virus that is believed to cause Infectious Mononucleosis (glandular fever).

ENDOCRINE: Pertaining to specific organs, or the complete system that secretes hormones into the circulation.

ERECTOR-SPINAE: The name applied to a group of muscles that extend along the length of the spine. As the name suggests, their main function is to keep the spine erect.

F

FIBROUS: Composed of, or containing fibres. Fibrous tissue is present in many different structures throughout the body. It is also formed in scar tissue during the natural healing process.

FIBROSITIS: An inflammatory condition affecting white fibrous tissue within chronically damaged muscle. The inflammation is combined with an increase in the volume of the tissue to cause a very tight, enlarged and tender area. The shoulders are the most common site for fibrositis to occur.

FORAMEN: An opening or hole, ususally found in bone that forms a natural passageway.

FATTY ACID: An acid that contains only carbon, hydrogen and oxygen which combines with glycerine to form fat.

FUNCTIONAL ANATOMY: Anatomy as applied to the interaction between different structures of the body during any activity.

G

GALL-BLADDER: A small pear-shaped sac which lies beneath the liver. Its function is to store bile that is produced by the liver.

GANGLION: A bundle of nerve cell bodies that lie outside the brain and spinal cord. (Plural = ganglia).

GANGLIONATED: Structures that contain ganglia.

GANGLION IMPAR: The ganglion which unites the two sympathetic trunks. It is found in front of the coccyx.

GASTRO-INTESTINAL: Pertaining to the stomach and gut.

GENITALIA: The organs of reproduction.

H

HEPATITIS: Inflammation of the liver.

HERPES VIRUS: A large group of DNA viruses, which includes herpes simplex (cold sores) and herpes zoster (shingles).

HIGHER CENTRES: The controlling mechanisms of the central nervous system within the brain.

HOMEOPATHY: A system of medicine whereby a minute dose of the drug stimulates the body to fight the disorder from within. It is based on the philosophy of treating like with like.

HOMEOSTASIS: The ability of the body to keep all functions working in a state of dynamic equilibrium.

HORMONE: An internal secretion which produces a specific physiological action on a target organ.

HVT: A high velocity thrust. The manipulative technique that produces a speedy gapping of a joint, usually accompanied by a loud ‘crack’.

HYPERMOBILE: Abnormal increase of movement.

HYSTERECTOMY: The surgical removal of the uterus (the womb).

I

IMMUNE SYSTEM: The system in the body responsible for fighting infection and disease.

IMMUNOG;OBULIN: A type of animal protein which produces antibodies. It is used in combating disease processes.

IMPAR: Not paired.

IMPULSES: The electrochemical process that travels along nerve fibres.

INFLUENZA: The ‘flu’; an acute viral infection of the respiratory tract.

INHIBITORY DRUGS: Chemicals that interfere with the normal physiological mechanism.

INTERSPINAL NERVES: Nerves that pass between two segments of the spine.

INTERVERTEBRAL: Between two adjacent vertebrae. *See Discs, intervertebral*

INTRAMUSCULAR: Within a muscle.

INTRAVENOUS: Within a vein.

INVOLUNTARY MECHANISM: The mechanism of the flow of cerebro-spinal fluid from the cranium to the sacrum, and its influence on other tissues.

K

KYPHOSIS: The convex curvature of the spine when viewed from the side. The dorsal spine is said to be KYPHOTIC if its naturally convex curvature is abnormally exaggerated.

L

LACRIMAL: Pertaining to tears.

LATERAL: To the side; in a position further away from the midline of the body.

LESION: A damaged area of tissue.

LEVATOR SCAPULAE: A muscle that attaches to the shoulder-blade and the upper neck. Its function is to raise the shoulder-blade.

LIGAMENT: A strong band of fibrous tissue that holds bones together.

LOBE: A divided portion of an organ.

LORDOSIS: The concave curvature of part of the spine when viewed from the side.

LUMBAR: Pertaining to the region of the loins, i.e. the area of the back between the thorax and the pelvis.

M

MANIPULATION: The expert treatment of the body by the hands.

MAOIs: Mono amino oxidase inhibitors; A group of antidepressant drugs.

ME: Myalgic Encephalomyelitis; the British name for chronic fatigue syndrome.

MEDULLA: The innermost portion of a structure.

METABOLISM: The chemical and physical process by which the living body is maintained.

MONONUCLEAR: Containing only one nucleus.

MOTOR NEURONE: A nerve that supplies a skeletal muscle to stimulate motion.

MUSCULOSKELETAL: Pertaining to the muscles and skeleton.

MYELIN: The fatty substances surrounding part of particular nerve fibres (known as MYELINATED fibres).

N

NEUROCHEMICAL: Pertaining to the chemistry of the nervous system.

NEUROLOGIST: A specialist in disorders of the nervous system.

NEUROMUSCULAR-SKELETAL SYSTEM: The system in the body comprising of nerves, muscles and the skeleton.

NEURON: A nerve cell.

NEUROTRANSMITTER: A chemical which stimulates activity when released at nerve endings, either transmitting between two nerves or between nerves and target tissues.

NORADRENALINE (or Norepinephrine): A neurotransmitter substance which is released in the sympathetic nervous system, and some central nerve endings.

O

OLFACTORY: Pertaining to the sense of smell.

P

PALPITATION: An increased awareness of the heartbeat.

PANACEA: A remedy; A cure-all.

PARALYSIS: Total or partial loss of movement in the body.

PARASYMPATHETIC NERVES: Autonomic nerves that stem from the cranium and the sacral regions and have different functions to sympathetic nerves.

PATHOGENIC: Pertaining to any organism that causes a disease.

PECTORALS: The collective name for the muscles of the chest, i.e. the pectoralis major and minor.

PEPTIC: Pertaining to the juices of the stomach and digestion.

PHYSIOLOGIST: A specialist in physiology, the study of the functioning of the body.

PHYSIOLOGY: The science of the function of living organisms, and how the body works.

PLACEBO: The beneficial response to treatment due to the patient's belief in its value. Placebo drugs are inactive substances that are given to gratify the patient.

PLASMA: The fluid part of the blood.

PLEXUS: A network of nerves.

POSTERIOR: At, or towards the back.

POSTGANGLIONIC: Positioned after (distal to) a ganglion.

PREGANGLIONIC: Positioned before (proximal to) a ganglion.

PROLAPSE: The downward fall of part, or all of an organ.

PROXIMAL: Nearer to a particular point, (opposite of distal).

Q

QUADRICEPS: The large four-headed muscle in the front of the thigh. Its main function is to extend and straighten the knee joint. Its tendon contains the patella (the knee cap).

R

RAMI COMMUNICANTES: A branch that connects two nerves.

RAMUS: A branch.

RECEPTORS: Receivers of certain nervous or chemical stimuli. They are situated at the ends of particular sensory nerves and on cells.

REFLEX: The automatic reaction that occurs in response to nervous stimulation.

REFLEXOLOGY: An alternative system of diagnosis and therapy. It is based on reflex points in the foot that correspond to different parts of the body.

REMISSION: The lull or cessation of the symptoms of a disease.

RSI: Repetitive strain injury.

S

SACRUM: The wedge-shaped bone situated directly beneath the lumbar spine. It comprises of five sacral bones fused together.

SCAPULA: The shoulder blade. (Plural: scapulae.)

SHIATSU: A form of oriental massage which concentrates on acupuncture points in the body.

SOFT TISSUE: The term used to describe the structural and connective tissue that is not bone, e.g. muscles and ligaments.

SOLAR PLEXUS: The coeliac plexus; the sympathetic plexus situated behind the stomach. It supplies the internal organs of the abdomen.

SOMATIC: Pertaining to the body; pertaining to the body wall as opposed to the internal organs.

SYNAPSE: A junction between two nerve cells.

SYNDROME: A collection of different symptoms that occur together.

T

TENDON: A fibrous continuation of the muscle body. It attaches muscle to bone.

TENNIS ELBOW: Lateral epicondylitis; an inflammation of the common tendon of the extensor muscles of the forearm due to an overuse injury.

THORACIC: Pertaining to the thorax.

THORAX: The chest; the section of the body between the neck and the abdomen. It is enclosed by the rib cage.

TRAPEZIUS: A muscle that attaches the neck to the shoulder blade and the collar bone. Its main function is to raise the shoulder. (Plural: trapezii.)

V

VAGUS: The vagus nerve, the 10th cranial nerve, which has sensory, motor and parasympathetic fibres. It travels down from the head to supply structrures in the neck, thorax and abdomen.

VASOCONSTRICTION: A decrease in the diameter of the blood vessels.

VASODILATION: An increase in the diameter of the blood vessels.

VENTRAL: Towards the front (opposite of dorsal).

VENTRICLE: The term applied to a cavity or chamber in the brain or the heart.

VERTEBRA: The individual bones of the spinal column.

VISCERA: The large organs of the body, plural of viscus.

VISCERAL: Pertaining to viscera.

VITAMIN: A group of organic substances that occur mainly in small amounts in food, and which are vital for the healthy functioning of the body.

Index

U

V

W

Y

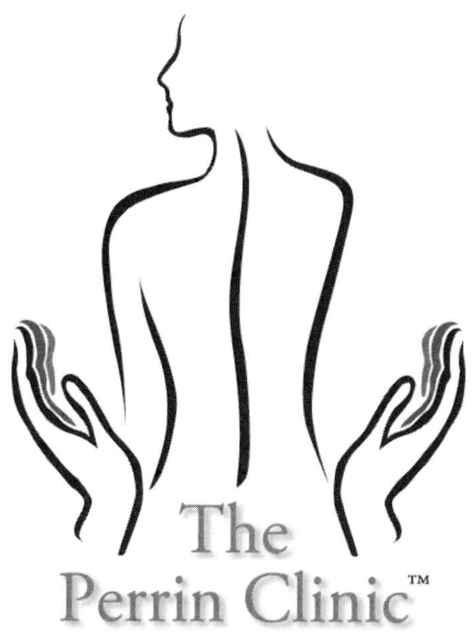

The Perrin Clinic is dedicated to helping all those with CFS/ME, using The Perrin technique™

The Perrin Clinic is also committed to training and monitoring practitioners who have been licensed to treat patients with The Perrin Technique™.

To find your nearest licensed practitioner visit:

www.theperrinclinic.com